EMILY MILLER

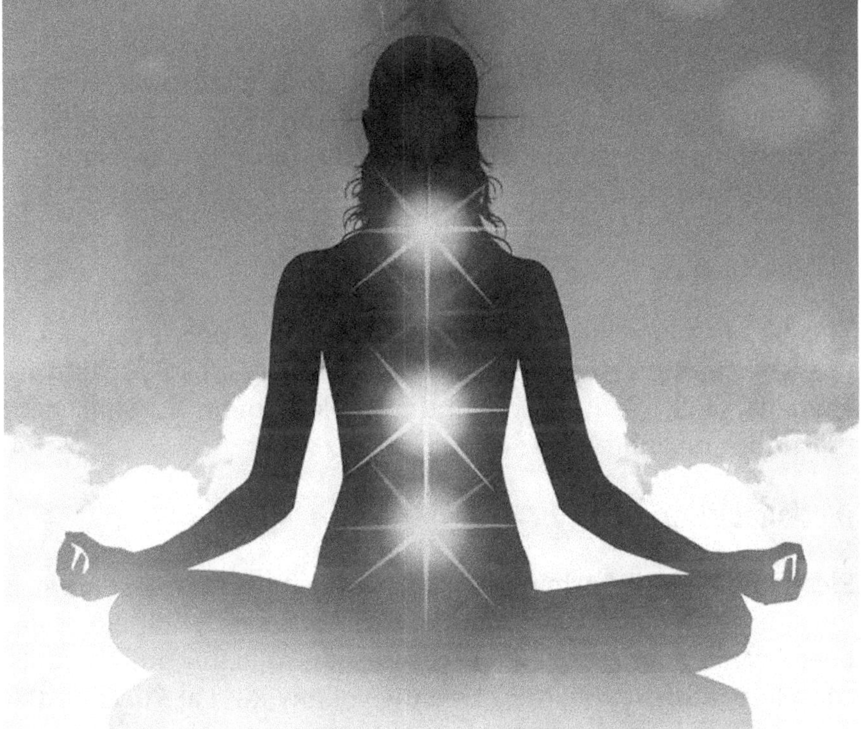

CHAKRAS
FOR BEGINNERS

THE ULTIMATE GUIDE TO HEALING YOUR CHAKRAS AND
BALANCING YOUR ENERGY THROUGH AWARENESS,
ESSENTIAL OILS, CRYSTALS AND YOGA. INCLUDING ALSO
SECRET TIPS FOR THIRD EYE AWAKENING

Chakras for Beginners

The ultimate guide to healing your chakras and balancing your energy through awareness, essential oils, crystals and yoga. Including also secret tips for third eye awakening.

Table of content

1. Introduction

Thank you for finding this book. I'm so honoured that it might help you in some way on your spiritual journey. In this book, my aim is to offer a comprehensive guide to the seven main chakras and to assist you in increasing your personal chakra awareness.

Throughout the book, I'll share with you a series of explanations and anecdotal illustrations, based on both personal experience and on fictional reconstructions inspired by experiences of chakra healing in my own healing practice. In this way, I hope to bring this area of study to life, so that you'll increase your understanding of how the chakra system operates and feel empowered with a basic understanding of some of the ideologies and principles involved in chakra healing.

Through these engaging stories, I also hope to illustrate the importance of our chakras in daily life - their influence on our circumstances, their impact on our thoughts and emotions, their ability to show us what's wrong and what needs to be fixed in our lives, from an energetic perspective. If you're an empath, you'll be pleased to learn tips for strengthening your solar plexus chakra and adopting new behaviours that will protect you from becoming drained and depleted in this area.

With the assistance of seven fictional characters and their stories, I'll show you how it feels when one of our chakras is blocked or out of balance, and give you tips and suggestions to heal the imbalances with meditation, crystals, essential oils and yoga.

I hope that by the end of this book you will have found answers to your most pressing questions about chakras and will feel ready to begin your own self-healing process.

At this time of incredible planetary change, as we go hurtling along the ascension timeline, incrementally creating heaven on earth, it wouldn't surprise me at all if you were reading this book because you've recently experienced a spiritual awakening and have found yourself asking some very big questions about your life. You might have read a lot of theory about chakras. You might have read some excellent teachings and philosophical discourses on Indian mysticism and chakra symbolism but feel no further forward in your own understanding of what's happening in your energy field or how to engage with it a way that's meaningful to you in a practical sense. At this point you might be longing for practical and lasting solutions to problems stemming from energy entanglement and psychic attack. You might be desperately looking for ways to feel grounded and strong in your physical body and your day to day reality.

Maybe you have recently experienced a disappointment or heartbreak and believe on some level that you're incapable of ever feeling happy again. You might even be experiencing physical symptoms that you intuitively know originate from something strange that's happening in your energy field or chakra system. *At this point, just a quick reminder that even if you are utterly convinced that this is the case, and that you are always 100 percent correct about your body and its workings, please consult a qualified medical professional if you're experiencing any unusual, persistent or worrying symptoms. At the time of writing this book, our world has become such a toxic place that it's a good idea to have a quick health check from time to time, to monitor the delicate balance of chemicals, hormones, vitamins and minerals in our bodies, as well as keeping up with any other important check-ups that might be relevant to you, personally. This book is in no way meant to be used as a tool for diagnosis or a substitute for proper medical advice and care.*

What you *will* find in this book, however, is information based on decades of personal study, research and experience. As an acutely sensitive empath, Reiki master, 5th dimensional energy practitioner and psychic development teacher, the experiences and tools I'll share with you in this book will be based on empirical, spiritual perspectives and vibrational phenomena. So, if you're looking for a dense text book on the history and science of the chakras, this might not be the book for you. This book is going to be packed with stories about the kinds of challenges faced by other sensitive spiritual seekers, and practical tools and tips for overcoming them.

I'm also not planning to share any brainy research written by clever scientific types, to somehow validate your experience as a spiritual being. Spiritual maturity means trusting yourself and the messages you receive through your clairsentient experience, your inner guidance and your team of angels and guides. With the escalation of spiritual and psychic awakenings currently occurring on the planet, the two most common problems I witness among those who are at the beginning of their spiritual journey are: an inability to get grounded, and problems with psychic attack or entanglement. If you picked this book up because you want to learn how to open, clear, heal and protect your chakras, I'm guessing you're probably not here to find out what a bunch of quantum physicists think about your Sahasrara.

Please don't misunderstand me; I think science is wonderful. Recent developments in science are a beautiful, powerful sign of our burgeoning desire to evolve spiritually, and future scientific discoveries will inevitably bring us back to a greater understanding of our spiritual essence. While quantum physics seems to leave us with more questions than answers, discoveries in string theory will ultimately prove what spiritual seekers have known all along: that we are made of light and we are all connected.

However, some of us currently find ourselves in a strange position: one of suddenly waking up to an understanding of our infinite connection to all things and beings (a 5th dimensional experience) while still swimming in the symptoms of separation– e.g. fear, greed, jealousy, anger, pain, envy etc. (3rd dimensional experiences). Because of these schisms and inconsistencies, you might feel bewildered as your energy bodies awaken in this 3D density, and you find yourself becoming more sensitive than ever. You might suddenly find it impossible to spend time in certain places or with certain, negative people. You might even be experiencing what feels like physical pain from deliberate psychic attacks, or from various *unconscious* forms of energetic intrusion. You might be feeling drained and depleted in a way that you just know within your heart has no scientific basis whatsoever - in the traditional sense. You might feel permanently exhausted and utterly frustrated to have had several doctors asking you never to darken their doorsteps again, or implying discreetly that you might be imagining things... because, in other words, there's just nothing (physically) wrong with you!

Maybe you know absolutely nothing about chakras but you've heard them talked about a lot and the word has stuck in your head, intuitively calling you to find out more. Even if you do already know a lot about chakras, you might find the following pragmatic, experience-based perspectives useful.

My personal intention is to share these tools with you in order to facilitate your highest and best next step along your path of spiritual awakening and to show you that chakra healing is not only possible but can also be life-changing!

2. What are Chakras?

We live in an energetic universe. Our experiences, thoughts, feelings, and even our physical health and well-being are all heavily influenced by the unseen energies within and around us. These energies and thoughts create matter, in the form of tangible ideas, health conditions and even many of the life circumstances from which we learn and grow.

As energy moves through the body, it is in a perpetual state of motion and is regulated, and processed by seven main wheel-like structures, or chakras, which keep this dynamic flow of life-force energy moving and circulating through the energy system in order to avoid an accumulation of toxic energy.

They absorb this energy, cleanse it and send it out into the energy bodies in order to feed them with appropriate quality of energy that will be uplifting, health-giving and life-enhancing.

The word chakra is derived from the Sanskrit word, cakra, which simply means 'wheel' or 'disc'. The chakras resonate at different vibrational frequencies, depending on their function and the area of life-experience to which they are related. For example, the lower chakras are more connected to our day-to-day existence and vibrate at a much lower and more tangible frequency.

They allow us to fulfil our earthly needs and everything we need in order to manifest fulfilling lives on the material plane, for example, food, shelter, security and financial stability (root chakra), creativity, sexuality/reproduction (sacral chakra) and personal power (solar plexus chakra), whereas, the upper chakras are more connected to our emotions and spiritual development.

Each chakra absorbs from the spectrum, the colour that is most resonant with its own level of vibration and function, and feeds this colour/vibration back into the energy system through a complex circuitry of energy channels, known as nadis, in order to facilitate the optimal health and wellbeing of each individual. If one or more of the chakras is blocked or out of balance, our mental, emotional and physical health will suffer.

The Root Chakra

For example, the first chakra - the root chakra (sometimes called the base chakra) is situated at the base of the spine and is the chakra which is most connected to our physical lives on Earth. This chakra vibrates at the same vibrational frequency as the colour red, and, therefore, absorbs this colour in order to give us the courage, strength and grounding to take care of our earthly survival needs and feel balanced and connected to our Earthly lives.

The root chakra governs and sends vitality to the hips, legs, bowels, intestines and adrenal glands – the body parts and organs related to movement, survival, fight or flight mechanisms and, in general, our ability to survive on Earth.

When the root chakra is healthy, balanced and spinning effectively, we feel at peace with our physical existence and able to meet our basic survival needs with ease. There are no major issues with money or with finding a nice home and if problems do arise in these areas, we are able to handle them with grace and without panic or fear. When the root chakra is in balance, we feel at home in our bodies and perfectly able to find enjoyment in the things of this world.

When the root chakra is blocked or not functioning correctly, we struggle to feel safe in the world and to meet our survival needs with ease. We may feel anxious, spaced out and somewhat detached from our physical and material lives. We might also experience lower back pain, stiffness in the hips and legs, or even problems in the reproductive areas of the body.

This chakra is thought to be related to the planets Earth, Saturn and Pluto (Experience, karmic lessons and cycles of birth, death and rebirth).

The Sacral Chakra

The second chakra, the sacral chakra, vibrates at the same frequency as the colour orange and relates to our ability to be creative and to enjoy expressing our sexuality and sensuality. While the root chakra supports us in creating a fulfilling material life, the sacral chakra supports our ability to enjoy the life we create. This chakra is located below the navel and governs the bladder, ovaries, testes and all reproductive functions.

This chakra is thought to be related to The Moon and Pluto (emotions, feeling, birth, death, rebirth and transformation – karmic cycles).

When the sacral chakra is healthy and functioning correctly, we feel creative and happy to be alive. We feel connected to the more passionate side of our nature and able to express our sexuality in appropriate ways. We feel connected to our bodies and enjoy feeding, clothing them and derive pleasure from the fruits of physical existence.

When this chakra is blocked or out of balance, there may be a reluctance to be creative and an inability to enjoy life. We may feel overwhelmed by work routines and cut off from our creativity and passion. In some cases, there may be a tendency to compensate for a lack of vitality and vibrancy with the use of stimulants such as coffee and other intoxicants. In extreme cases, dysfunctions of the sacral chakra can lead to addictive behaviours.

The Solar Plexus Chakra

The third chakra, the solar plexus chakra, vibrates at the same frequency as the colour yellow and is related to our personal power, intuitive knowing (gut feelings) and our ability to develop healthy levels of self-esteem, wisdom and confidence in our abilities. It is at this level that we begin to reflect on life and observe it, rather than simply surviving or enjoying it. We ascend in awareness and evolve into *psychic* beings who are able to discern the qualities of the energies around us.

The solar plexus chakra has been referred to as the psychic brain, and it is one of the most important centres for developing intuition. When we are able to connect with this centre and follow our gut feelings, we develop wisdom and greater self-awareness. This chakra is located above the navel but below the rib cage and governs the stomach, digestive organs and nervous system.

If the solar plexus is blocked or is not functioning correctly, we feel a lack of self esteem and an inability to respond authentically to the energies we experience in the world. When this chakra (our centre of personal power) is compromised, we might feel controlled or manipulated by others. We might feel disempowered and out of touch with our truest will and desires. On the physical level we might experience stomach issues, digestive complaints or nervous conditions that stem from not trusting our own gut instincts and following our true path in life. Within the stomach, we register our first responses to energy, our gut feelings, butterflies or clenching, and of course our nervous system becomes tense when we're exposed to too much unsettling energy for too long.

This chakra also governs the liver and the spleen, which are also related to the many ways our bodies react to the people and situations around us. The spleen reminds us to look for the natural sweetness in life, and when we feel drained by others, our first impulse is to replace lost vital energies through the unhealthy use of sugar and comfort foods. The liver is where we hold most of our anger at an energetic level.

This chakra is thought to be related to the planets the Sun, Mars and Mercury (selfhood, force of will and communication).

The Heart Chakra

The fourth chakra is the heart chakra, which vibrates at the same frequency as deep, forest green. This is the centre that allows us to feel love and compassion for others and to process our emotions in healthy ways. Through a healthy heart chakra, we become able to express our feelings and sustain healthy, loving connections and intimate relationships with others. This chakra is located at the centre of the chest and governs the healthy functioning of the physical heart, chest, lungs and thymus gland. This chakra is thought to be related to the planets Venus and Earth (manifesting love on the physical plane).

If the heart chakra is not functioning correctly, we feel cut off emotionally and may seek to isolate ourselves from others. Love feels unsafe and it seems easier to become cynical about relationships and avoid them altogether. It's interesting to note that the Sanskrit name for the heart chakra is anahata which means unwounded, intact, unhurt, unbeaten. (Please see the Chakra Colours and Functions Chart below for the Sanskrit names of all seven chakras). This implies that a healthy heart chakra is one that is 'like new', full of innocence and wonder; it is like a heart that has never been hurt before and which, therefore, feels safe, open and receptive.

If the heart chakra is overactive, we tend to give too much of ourselves and make unwise choices in love – giving our time and devotion to those who don't truly value us or the love we bring. When we bring the heart chakra back into balance, we make wiser, more loving (and self-loving) choices, and all our relationships flourish and feel good.

The Throat Chakra

The fifth chakra is the throat chakra, which vibrates at the same frequency as the colour blue and relates to our ability to find a voice in the world and to express ourselves truthfully and with pure intention. A healthy throat chakra supports us in expressing our true inner essence in the world and is, therefore, also connected to finding our true purpose in life.

The throat chakra is also related to our ability (or inability) to speak up for ourselves. Essentially, the throat chakra supports us in our ability to be ourselves more fully and to communicate our truth with purity, love, compassion and clarity.

Physically, this chakra rules the thyroid, tonsils, throat, neck and shoulders. It is located between the collar bones, over the physical throat area.

This chakra is thought to be related to the moon and Venus (expressions of emotion, love and beauty).

If the throat chakra is blocked or functioning incorrectly, we find it hard to share our true feelings or to truly be ourselves in the world. We may have problems with expressing our thoughts and feelings publicly, and in taking the necessary steps to break out of unhealthy work situations in order to follow our true calling in life. We may experience persistent problems with throat complaints, stiffness in the neck and shoulders and even digestive issues (the result of constantly swallowing our true feelings). If the throat chakra is overactive, we may find ourselves speaking inappropriately or speaking over others, desperate to get our point across because we feel generally unheard.

When the throat chakra is healthy, we are able to speak and listen with compassion and find the kindest and wisest words in every situation – words that will inspire others to become their greatest selves.

The Third Eye Chakra

The sixth chakra is the third eye chakra, which is related to our sixth sense and our ability to use our extra sensory perception and psychic faculties to receive psychic information and guidance. This chakra vibrates on the same frequency as the colour indigo and is located between and slightly above the physical eyes.

When this chakra is healthy, we are able to receive psychic information to guide our lives more wisely and with more insight. In a more practical sense, when the third eye is balanced, we are able to see the truth with our inner vision, and with the support of this chakra we can see into a range of possible futures and make informed choices, based on our ability to predict the events that might follow a particular action. This, in turn, allows us to make wiser choices, as we make plans and dream dreams for the future.

This chakra governs the physical eyes, sinuses, head, pituitary and pineal gland. The effective functioning of these glands is essential for the effective functioning of our inner and outer vision.

This chakra is thought to be related to the planets Neptune and Jupiter (psychic ability and expansion).

If the third eye chakra is blocked or functioning incorrectly, we may lose our sense of purpose and direction, and feel unable to connect with our inner wisdom. Psychic faculties will be limited or impaired and we may feel a sense of spiritual disconnection. In extreme cases, there may also be problems with headaches, blocked sinuses and fogginess or dizziness.

The Crown Chakra

The seventh chakra is the crown chakra which is located at the top of the head and vibrates at the same frequencies as the colours violet and white. Often described as the thousand petal lotus, this chakra is the seat of our ability to connect with the God of our understanding and to transcend the human condition. This chakra is the one which is the most mysterious and perhaps misunderstood. It is the chakra through which we go beyond ourselves, into the unknown and the indescribable.

The time honoured way to achieve balance in the crown chakra is to develop a daily practice of meditation, yoga, chanting or any other spiritual practice that allows us to switch off the mind and journey into the silent stillness. The crown chakra is a gateway to heaven, or what the Buddhist call Nirvana. It is the chakra through which we experience the unknown and embrace the unknowable.

This chakra governs the brain, skull, skin and hypothalamus. When this chakra is healthy and balanced, we feel a connection with all other beings and are able to extend compassion towards everyone, because we see the bigger picture and the higher plan in everything. If you wish to connect with guides, angels and ascended masters, or receive inspired and channelled guidance, developing this chakra will connect you with higher sources of guidance and wisdom.

This chakra is thought to be related to the planets Uranus and Mercury (innovation, change and communication).

If the crown chakra is blocked, we may feel cut off spiritually and unable to believe in anything beyond the physical realm. We may feel forgotten or abandoned by God and have no sense of connection with those who love and guide us from the spirit realms. In extreme cases, there may be headaches, migraines, insomnia, faithlessness and irritability.

Please see the Chakra Colours and Functions Chart below, for an at-a-glance reference to all the essential chakra information shared in this chapter.

3. Chakra Balancing and Alignment

Further on in this book, you'll find, at the end of each anecdotal chapter on the individual chakras, a meditation to increase the health and well-being the chakra described in the story. These meditations are extremely effective if used consistently. Over time, you'll find your chakras becoming stronger and more able to support you in your desire to enrich every area of your life.

In order to bring the chakras into balance and alignment with each other, we practice drawing energy up from the earth, through the feet and the lower chakras. The more we visualise this energy travelling up from mother earth to support us, the more empowered we become to enjoy all that life has to offer. When the lower chakras are in alignment with each other, we feel a greater connection with the earth, and our material existence is greatly enriched. This dynamic flow of life-force energy is known as the liberation current, because by drawing this sacred earth energy up into the heart, we liberate ourselves from living purely at the base level of survival, and connect with our hearts and our higher spiritual potential.

As we visualise the energy moving up from the earth, through the lower chakras and into the heart chakra, we can also draw energy down from the heavens, through the crown, third eye and throat chakras. This energy allows us to balance the upper chakras, in order to enrich our spiritual lives. This divine life-force energy (known as the manifestation current) pours down through our chakras of inspiration, inner vision and pure expression until it flows into the heart chakra and combines with the liberation current, connecting heaven and earth within our hearts and ensuring that we move towards balance (and eventually mastery) in all areas of life, while focusing our intentions on love.

The energy that flows from above is known as the manifestation current, because through it, we manifest our dreams, visions and desires onto the earth plane. It is through this current that we bring Heaven to Earth and make our dreams a reality, as we imagine, visualise and then speak them into existence.

Both currents are essential: we need the liberation current to bring balance to our material lives, so that we can experience rich and fulfilling physical lives. We need the manifestation current to connect us to the higher spiritual planes, so that our lives have greater depth and spiritual meaning.

In recent years, I have been guiding my students to visualise drawing the liberation current up from the centre of the new Earth, with its ascended crystalline structure and new ascension template. Experiment with these visualisations and see what works best for you.

4. How the Chakras Operate

Whether we know it or not, we exist in several dimensions at once. These include dimensions of thought, feeling, emotion, telepathy, intellect, pure energy, cosmos, causality, light and astral potentiality.

As much as we sometimes imagine that the chair we're sitting on and the desk upon which we rest our technological devises are the only realities that exist, we are far greater, more expanded and more creative than we can even begin to imagine.

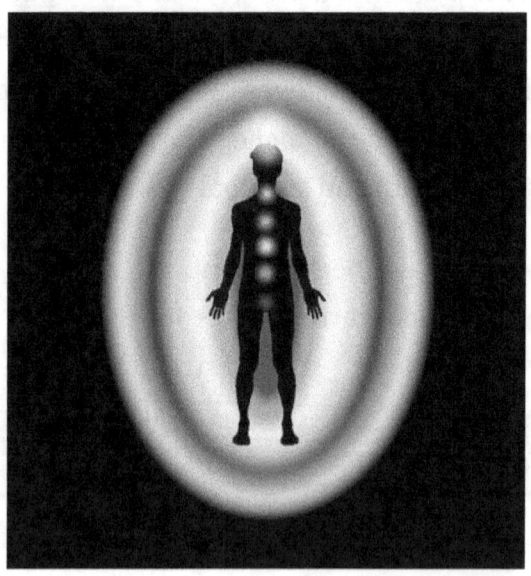

For each plane of experience that exists, we each have a body that enables us to travel, explore and experience events and possibilities within the corresponding plane of existence. For example, we have a physical body for the purpose of exploring life on the physical plane, an emotional body with which we journey through the world of emotions, a light body through which we experience the potential for ascending into a state of pure bliss and unconditional love, an astral body through which we experience parallel and potential timelines, and a range of other phenomena which are lived out during what we call "dreams, imaginings and projections".

Through a network of chakras and nadis, each of the bodies is able to receive, process and feed energy to the entire energy system. In the case of the material plane, energy is taken in through food, to feed the physical body and ensure its efficient functioning in the 3rd dimension. The body takes the food in through the mouth and, through the various digestive processes, extracts the nutrients that are useful and discards the rest. Depending on the quality of the food we consume, the body will either have access to very high-quality nutrition or barely adequate sustenance. Depending on what we feed it with, the body will, over time, become supple, strong and full of health and vitality or sluggish, blocked and inflexible.

Similarly, if we grew up in a toxic environment with abusive or neglectful parents and continued to experience abusive relationship cycles throughout our lives, our emotional bodies would be sluggish and overburdened with toxic, stagnant and possibly repressed emotions. Rage, regret, resentment, self-loathing and heartbreak can all be seen in the heart chakra as they manifest themselves into dark thought forms in this area.

As with food, if the emotional sustenance available has always been of a very low quality, the emotional body will struggle to be fit and healthy and the heart chakra itself will become stagnant and full of unprocessed emotion, like waste food matter languishing in the stomach of a junk food addict. Only, in the case of an over-stuffed heart chakra, instead of feeling fat, sick and lethargic, we might simply feel very guarded, insular, reclusive and unwilling to trust new people or embrace new encounters.

When the heart chakra is blocked, we become emotionally constipated. We might often feel and know there are some tears we need to cry. In fact, we might often feel as if we are on the brink of tears, but for some reason they just won't come out. When the tears do eventually start to flow, we know in our hearts that the healing has begun.

In the process of consuming and digesting food, pranic (life force) energy is also produced and passed along into the unseen energy system. The higher the vibration of the food we consume, the more the other (unseen energy) bodies are recharged and healed by this input from the third dimension. The nature of the chakras and the energy bodies is relational rather than unique and isolated. In other words, everything feeds everything else.

As well as the main chakras, within each of our energy bodies there is a system of smaller chakras and wheels within wheels, which enable us to keep our energetic system functioning optimally - a series of cogs that interconnect and cooperate in order to clean and recycle energy as it runs through each body.

Through the seven main chakras, we each maintain a meaningful, spiritual connection to our physical bodies, and process the many life experiences and lessons we encounter in this exciting manifesting experiment called *life on Earth*. In this way, we are constantly collecting and collating the sum of these experiential parts that we may consciously or unconsciously gain access to on our journey through the many dimensions in which we concurrently exist.

The crown chakra connects our physical body to the higher realms and draws on sustenance from their purified spaces, from the higher self, from our guides and angelic teachers and from our soul families.

The crown chakra and the light body act as receivers of vital information from the mother ship – God, the higher self, soul groups, guides and teachers - as well as allowing us to understand, process and utilise the energy that's sent to us from others - intentionally or unintentionally, kindly and lovingly or immaturely and malevolently. When we learn how to connect with energy and light from our divine origins and channel it intentionally, this energy also feeds the physical body, keeping it ageless, vital and radiant. We process this vital life force energy through all our energy bodies, and the energy processing and recycling centres for this energy are the chakras.

Each wheel is connected through a network of energy threads and, through very similar threads, we are all connected to every other being, for better or worse. Through this powerful network, we receive and discern the quality of energy that comes into our field from others, and unconsciously decide whether an incoming energy is in vibrational harmony with our highest spiritual aspirations at any given time.

In my experience as a healer, just like our very electrical and dynamic brains, each of our chakras is able to think, listen, record, speak and create. Through our chakras we are constantly inhaling and exhaling the universe, creating and un-creating the world as we know it, in a never ending divine manifesting meditation that springs from our need (root chakra) our desire (sacral) our craving (solar plexus) our love (heart) our desire to express our truest self (throat) our unrealised vision (3rd eye) and our knowledge that we are love, we are all one and we will only find peace when we recognise that we are all connected (crown).

Please see the table below for an overview of the chakras and their functions, including their Sanskrit names. For each chakra, practice saying these mystical names out loud as you meditate on each one and see how this affects your vibration – just notice what you feel!

My wish for this book is that you'll feel able to experience it to some extent, rather than simply reading it. I want it to take you on a journey into, through and ultimately beyond yourself, because I believe that's what you're here for, and you know in your heart that chakra awareness can only be experienced in one way - vibrationally. If it were possible to learn everything you needed to learn from simply reading words in your head, you wouldn't be reading yet another book; you would have already learned.

5. Chakra Colours and Functions Chart

Chakra Name	Physical body parts governed by chakra	Position	Functions	Colours
Root Chakra **Muladhara**	Hips, legs, bowels, intestines and adrenal glands	Base of the spine	Grounding, security, feeling safe, strength and wisdom to meet our survival needs, independence, balance, material abundance	Red
Sacral Chakra **Swadhisthana**	The bladder, ovaries, testes and all reproductive functions	Below the navel	Creativity, joy, sexuality, pleasure, appetite, desire	Orange
Solar Plexus Chakra **Manipura**	Stomach, digestive organs and nervous system, liver and spleen	Above the navel, below the ribcage	Wisdom, personal power, self-esteem, self-determination, will power, psychic hunches	Yellow & Gold
Heart Chakra **Anahata**	Heart, chest, lungs and thymus gland	Centre of the chest	Love, compassion, contentment, kindness, connection	Deep green & Pink
Throat Chakra **Vishuddha**	Thyroid, tonsils, throat, neck and shoulders	The throat	Communication, confidence, self-expression, eloquence, fluency	Cornflower Blue
Third Eye Chakra **(Ajna)**	the physical eyes, sinuses, head, pituitary and pineal gland	Centre of the forehead	Inner vision, clarity, clairvoyance, psychic ability	Indigo & purple
Crown Chakra **(Sahasrara)**	The brain, skull, skin and hypothalamus	The top of the head	Self-realisation, spirit, higher consciousness, communion with God, angels and non-physical guides and masters	Violet & white

6. The Chakras and Human Evolution

Currently on our planet, we are in the midst of incredible transformation – a co-creation that has been several decades in the making. When a cry for peace leaves the heart chakra, it speaks to the environment, sending ripples of love out into the quantum field and beginning a process of ascension into pure consciousness. This is the process that has been catalysed by the many light-workers who came before us, and because of their loving intentions, and the quantity of high-frequency energy they were capable of moving through their bodies, chakras and energy fields, we are on the cusp of an unstoppable evolution in collective, human consciousness.

As we move through the world, consciously or unconsciously, we are also creating our experience. Chakras, full of energy colour and light are constantly moving, swelling and growing. They absorb light and transform it into the colour that is most needed. (Please see the table above for an overview of the corresponding colours for each chakra).

So, if we imagine that energy is light-food for all our bodies, including the physical, 3D body, the chakras could almost be seen as the mouth and the digestive organs for each body, and colours could be viewed as the specific nutrients needed for the optimal functioning of each of those organs. For example, the skin uses vitamins A, D, C, and E to keep in healed, self-repairing, self-regenerating, radiant, effective and supple. The root chakra uses the colour red to keep us grounded, strong, connected and capable of meeting our abundant earthly needs.

In a symphonic cacophony of activity, depending on our consciousness, our company and our environment, the chakras are constantly opening and closing, stopping and starting, inhaling and exhaling, sifting and sorting, writing and rewriting, pulsating and contracting, rising and falling vibrating and spinning, swirling and reaching, always listening always speaking, resting and dancing, discerning and feeling, intuiting and healing, warning and honing, and informing us of how to navigate an infinite number of encounters, dimensions, people and possibilities, constantly seeking balance.

Those of us who perceive life as an eternal continuum of pre-birth, birth, life, death and rebirth, and who believe we have come from another place *into* a lifespan on Earth, may often imagine that when we arrive here on Earth, we leave behind a glorious heaven to which we will one day return when we have completed our tour of duty and can finally return to paradise. However, at this time of unprecedented growth and awakening of human consciousness, there might be a more exciting perspective for us to consider: rather than leaving heaven behind and stoically taking on a new physical body each time we incarnate, perhaps we are here to create heaven on earth through our joyful, inhaling, exhaling, dancing, singing, swelling, swirling, glittering, pulsating, living, loving, breathing engagement with the earth, through our dynamic energy systems and chakras. Heaven is alive and well within each one of us, potentially making our lives a paradise, if we take the time to take care of our energetic health and our divine connection with our divine mother earth.

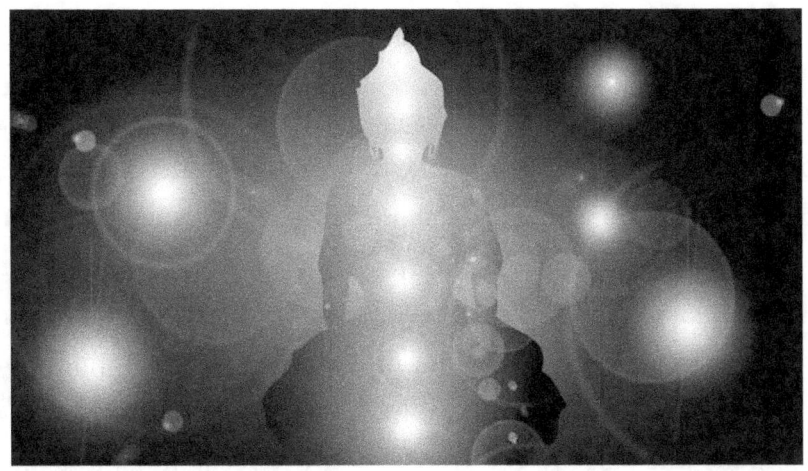

Surely, this is the legacy we have inherited from centuries of yogis and gurus, eons of Buddhas, Buddhists and bodhisattvas, all meditating and chanting for the upliftment of humanity and the highest good of all. Decades, maybe centuries of old-school spiritualists, light workers and pioneers in the field of energy medicine, all bringing their deep love and compassion for humanity, has brought us to this tipping point. They all knew this time was coming, and to speak about chakras or any other consciousness-raising energy phenomenon without mentioning our current ascension would just be weird. #elephantintheroom

7. The Interrelated Nature of Chakras

When I'm working with a healing client, one of the first things I notice is which of their chakras feels the most constricted, blocked or under attack. When I have finished clearing and healing the compromised chakras, I often spend time balancing and aligning all 7 chakras. Somewhere in this mysterious healing process, I'm often struck by not only the power and influence of the chakras over the mental, emotional and physical health of the client but also by the interaction *between* them, and their interdependence in creating a fully-functioning and holistically healthy human being.

For example, there was once a client who came to me to work on psychic and intuitive development. She'd been feeling and sensing her angels and guides around her and wanted to know how to open up and close down safely so that she could begin to see and hear them better. However, her heart had been so thoroughly broken by a series of disappointments and bereavements, that it was impossible for her to become grounded enough to even begin practicing psychic work of a high quality. So, before we could start work on opening up her third eye, we had to work on moving the energy through a large blockage in her heart and down into the lower chakras where she had been resisting becoming fully grounded.

It's interesting to note that in many cases, I've had to work the hardest on grounding with people who don't really feel particularly happy about their lives here on Earth, and the more I worked with this client, let's call her, Brenda, the more I noticed that she was wasn't particularly happy about being in a physical body. When we first began our sessions, she had actually been taking antidepressants for over twenty years, but after several months of focused and committed work on opening, clearing and repairing her heart chakra she was able to heal from her grief and later reported to me that she had had several heart-opening spiritual awakenings and, with support and guidance from her GP) had stopped taking her medication. As a result of this heart opening, we were finally able to begin moving the energy through to her feet so that she could get fully grounded. Brenda's story shows us, once again, that there is indeed a powerful connection between all the chakras and that they work most effectively when they are perfectly balanced, aligned with each-other and rotating and moving together in harmony.

Imagine for a second the cogs you might see if you examine the inner workings of a machine. Each cog is necessary for the effective overall functioning of the machine. If one tiny cog becomes blocked, stuck, sticky, rusty or simply breaks down and refuses to co-operate with the others, the functioning of the entire organism is impaired. Although in this book we will be focusing mainly on the seven main chakras, when I allow myself to become aware of the entire multidimensional chakra system, I often sense that the picture below offers a much closer approximation of what's happening.

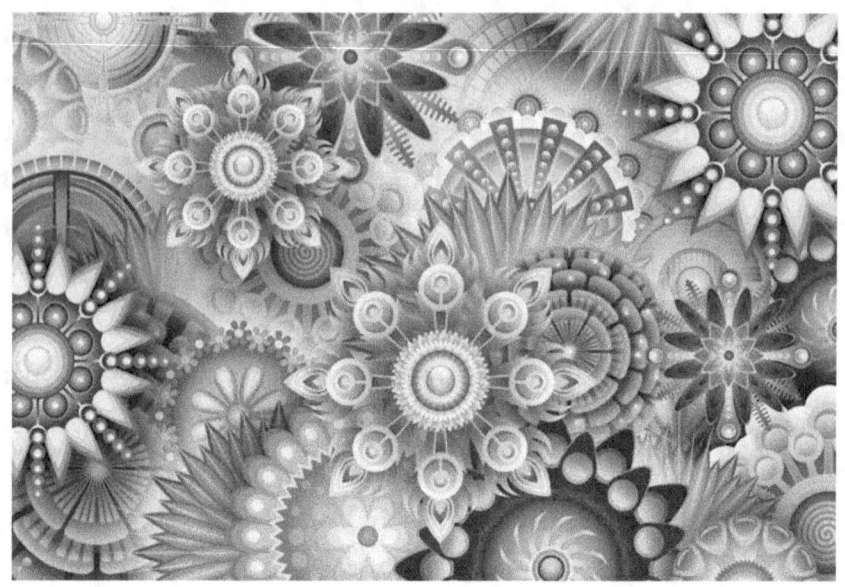

When we think of the seven main chakras – the ones we most commonly describe as being held within the physical body, we see an image of the seven main energy centres stacked up within the body in vertical alignment. When we think about how divine life-force energy is drawn down into the body, through the crown chakra, and up through the root chakra, it's sometimes useful to have an image of all chakras, front and back, attached to the pranic tube, through which they are all fed with light. Through this tubular structure - which extends from far above the crown (and into the heavens) and far below the feet (grounding us into the new earth grids) our entire chakra system receives vital divine energy from heaven and earth.

This powerful image works well for our chakra alignment meditations, and it's useful to keep them in mind when we imagine or intend that there is a dynamic flow of essential life force energy moving through and between these powerful centres, unhindered and unrestricted. When we are able to become proficient in moving energy through these centres, balancing, aligning, opening and closing them at will, we become truly empowered beings who are able to safely awaken our psychic awareness, shield, protect and heal ourselves from encounters with negativity, heal our precious world, and become the divine beings we know ourselves to be.

Something that is now fairly commonly discussed is the idea that there are actually at least 12 chakras, which become visible when we are able to perceive those that extend beyond the physical body, both above and below.+

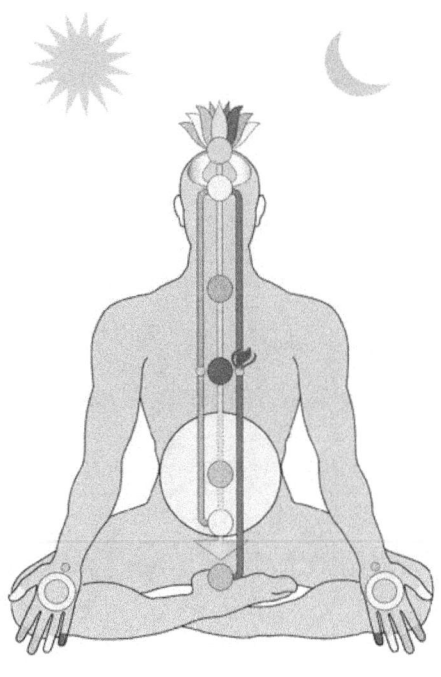

Aside from the full chakra template, there are also several smaller chakras situated throughout our entire bodies. There are chakras in our hands, feet, ears, eyes (and at many other receptive sites), that we very rarely speak of. There are chakras connecting us to the earth and to the heavens, to our parents, our children and our ancestors.

8. The Importance of Wheels

We only need to look around us to see the importance of wheels in allowing the efficient functioning of our daily lives. Wheels allow us to travel on buses and in cars. Wheels allow us to transport food and other essentials to wherever they are needed. Wheels keep our physical world in motion, and chakras keep divine light flowing and circulating through our hearts, minds and bodies and functioning optimally throughout our journey of incarnation and beyond.

Even in the afterlife, chakras and other kinds of energy vertices are necessary as the glue between many possibilities, and as long as we have the need for a physical body, our chakras operate as a series of integration points – a kind of spirit/body interface.

Take your time discovering and working with these energies and, where possible, find an experienced and ethical teacher to work with – one who practices good energy-shielding and clearing techniques and who can guide your development, not only from a place of knowledge and education but also from a place of psychic insight and personal experience.

9. Chakras and the Physical Body

In my work as a healer, I have often seen heaviness and blockages in the sacral chakra only to have a client confirm that there have been health issues in the reproductive organs. I have seen many blocked heart chakras in the case of clients who later revealed that they had suffered with conditions such as asthma, heart palpitations and a variety of other heart and chest related conditions. I have also seen many blocked throat chakras in clients who revealed or confirmed life-long issues with throat complaints.

For the purpose of this book, I'll be focusing on the area of work with which I have gained the most experience over the years - the clearing and balancing of energy for mental and emotional wellbeing, grounding and clarity in spiritual development. In my humble opinion and in my experience of working directly with clients, this is the fundamental approach that has been the most meaningful and effective in improving all conditions, including those of overall health and life circumstances.

When we focus on a holistic view of health and happiness, it is perhaps more empowering to view health as a state of vibrational awareness rather than applying 'disease or no disease' philosophy. Perhaps in the future it will be recognised that committing to a regular practice of clearing and balancing our chakras and our entire energy system is one of the most empowering things we can do to achieve and maintain optimal health. As many of us are now aware, most physical complaints that develop in our bodies were manifested energetically long before they appeared as physical disease and the overall resolution of long-term conditions may, therefore, be found somewhere at a vibrational root cause.

However, these karmic wounds and patterns are often very deeply ingrained, and although chakra healing and balancing has been known to ease symptoms in many cases, it is always best to bring your physical complaints to a medical practitioner to ensure that you receive correct and appropriate treatment, whilst also working to strengthen the energy field.

10. Why are Chakras Important?

Think of each of your chakras as a mini brain that collects, and records into its database, information of a specific quality, for better or worse. This allows you to save, process, understand and retrieve when needed, memories of your experiences in several different areas of experience. Your chakras are a kind of living, breathing, organic, multidimensional classroom.

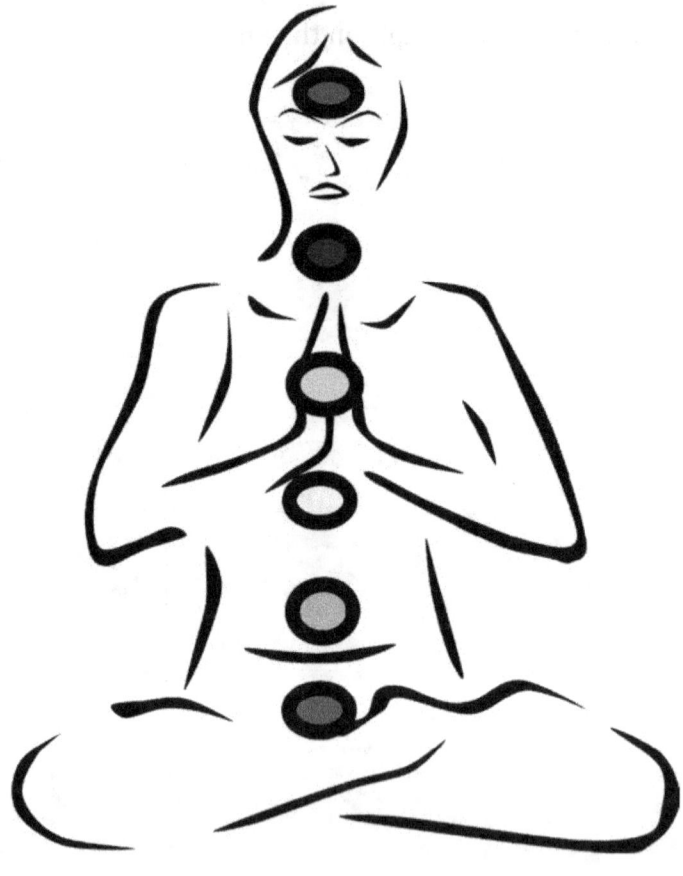

Imagine, for example, that you have been brought up in an emotionally abusive family.

Your root, solar plexus and heart chakras will be carrying saved recordings of survival strategies, unpleasant thoughts about yourself, protection against manipulation, repressed rage and desperation. Every abusive word that was ever spoken to you will have been recorded throughout your chakra system, where feelings of unworthiness continue to fester and grow with each added insult. Even you ear chakras will have suffered as a result of listening to insults, tantrums and other kinds of aural violence. In your third eye chakra, your vision may be cloudy, and distorted by images of your abusers, which prevent you from ever seeing a bright future or having faith in your visions of a more hopeful future.

As an adult, many years after leaving the emotionally abusive home, you might wonder how, even after years of therapy, you still seem to be repeatedly attracting the same kinds of people, situations and experiences – those which reinforce for you, again and again, every miserable insult or accusation that was every thrown at you in those abusive formative years.

This is where we need to look deeper, to discover the energetic imprints that have been recorded, year after year (sometimes for decades) and inscribed into your very being, causing you to emit their frequency out into the world for all to feel. You might as well be wearing a tee shirt that says all the things your chakras are screaming out into the energetic biosphere, because whether you consciously believe them or not, they are inscribed upon your very being.

Energy imprints can be like fingerprints - they are unique and uniquely identifying. Your lips maybe moving and saying "I'm amazing at my job and deserve to be rewarded appropriately", but if your chakras are screaming "I'll take much less than I deserve because I fundamentally dislike myself!"the world will be obedient - until you erase the program and write a new one. It's just a story – usually someone else's - and it can be rewritten.

These unproductive messages that we have accepted into our chakras are also constantly sending messages through our entire body systems, feeding us with a set of ideas that give us a kind of template for being. Simply put, these ideas tell us who we are. If you're not this, then you must be that. If you're not that, then you must be this. We must all be something. We all need to have something to work on, to adjust, to grow from and grow into. I recently heard someone say, "If you live on Earth school, you have a human curriculum; no one is exempt."

Finding out what's written on your charkas and setting your intention to write a new story can be powerful, not only in terms of our physical healing but also in enabling us to gradually improve our life conditions and circumstances.

Whenever we feel a lack of interest in life and in our surroundings, clearing the sacral chakra can help us to feel inspired again. When we are lacking vision and feeling hopeless about the future, clearing the third eye chakra can enable us to see a brighter future and detach ourselves from other people's imprints and intentions for us. When we are acutely sensitive to our environment and the energies swimming around in the collective, clearing these upper chakras can help us to become more aware of our own path and reawaken our connection with our guides and non-physical teachers.

The next time you suddenly feel depressed or confused, ask yourself, *Is this energy mine? Does it truly belong to me?* And if not, *how can I clear it and return to a state of wholeness, peace and balance.* Close your eyes, sit in a nice relaxed and comfortable position and visualise white light pouring in through the top of your head, clearing away all doubt, negativity and uncertainty.

11. Psychic Development and the Chakras

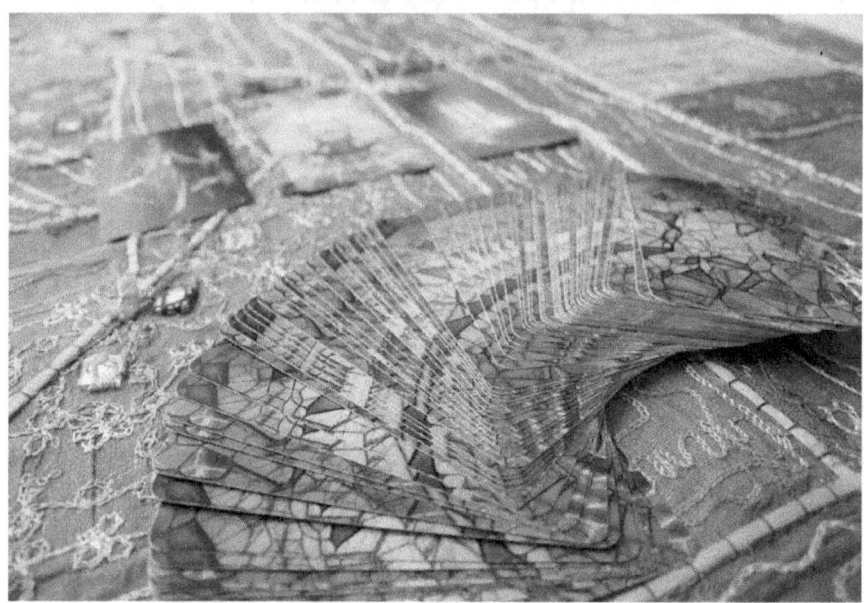

This is an area that is as vast as it is fascinating, and we can no more underestimate the importance of the chakras in psychic development than that of our guides, angels and non-physical teachers.

Usually, when I begin teaching psychic development with a new student, the first thing I usually work on is grounding. In other words, opening up to divine energy and allowing it to flow through each of the chakras until it flows down into the root chakra and creates a strong grounding chord into the loving and sacred centre of the new Earth template.

As soon as the energy begins to flow through the chakras, I observe where it flows easily and where it becomes stuck or finds it difficult to penetrate effectively. I often see or sense cloudy areas in one or more of the chakras and work with the light and with the assistance of higher teachers, angels and guides to release anything that prevents the student from grounding.

Sometimes issues concerning self-expression are apparent in the throat chakra and, often, these issues will lead both myself and the student into other areas of discovery, such as past life wounding – for example in cases where these blockages were caused by physical past life traumas. On several occasions, I have worked on releasing karmic patterning which was formed by unpleasant death experiences, for example, experiences of persecution and torture. This is extremely common among light-workers, who have usually emerged in this lifetime from a long and chequered past which includes many lifetimes devoted to spreading spiritual truths. Often, their efforts were thwarted or punished in these lifetimes and they have returned to heal these wounds once and for all.

I often find that these ancient imprints, which can lead a student or client to feel unsafe in the world, are still engraved into the chakras several lifetimes later. Many of my clients are previously persecuted light-workers and spiritual seekers who now feel unworthy of being a spiritual messenger. There are often chords and attachments connected to their chakras, keeping them attached to the souls they believe they have wronged or let down in the past by being a poor leader. There have even been cases where those who have punished or even executed them in the past have remained connected to them and now require their forgiveness. When these wounds and attachments are released, all parties are free to continue along their respective spiritual paths and there is usually a visceral feeling of relief and release that runs through the energy field of everyone who participates in the healing session.

Often it is only when these attachments and blockages are released that the student can receive the full flow of life-force energy necessary for them to become the divine channels they wish to be. In many cases, it can take weeks of before they are free to allow this energy in and connect with their guides in a fully aligned and 5th dimensional way.

When we begin to prepare for 5th dimensional psychic and intuitive work, we must endeavour to prepare ourselves in a 5th dimensional way. This means that in order to become pure channels for the highest and truest spiritual insights available, we must clear our energies and our intentions daily. When we work hard to remain clear, awake, and aware, keeping a regular check on the quality of energy that runs through us, we increase our ability to rely on the purity of the information we receive through the heart, the third eye and the crown chakra. By increasing our discernment in this way, we can increasingly learn to trust the hunches and nudges we feel in our gut, at the level of the solar plexus, and as a result of this, when our psychic mechanisms form pictures in our minds to translate the energetic downloads we receive from Spirit, they will be filtered through a pure channel of higher spiritual understanding. In turn, this higher awareness gradually teaches us the difference between our human responses of fear and suspicion and the wise counsel from our guides and higher selves regarding the impact of the choices we make in our lives. It is only through a clear understanding of how to correctly evaluate the quality of energy that runs through our chakras that we can make sense of the unseen, energy-based realms and allow them to inform these choices.

It the crown chakra is clear and bright, I know that my student is ready to receive a very high frequency and prolific kind of inspiration from the divine. Perhaps they are writers or channels.

When I see or sense golden light around the solar plexus, I know that they will receive a higher vibration of gut knowing and intuition.

When the heart chakra is fully open and represented by symbols of purity, for example, white flowers or unique symbols from their guides, in gold or violet, I know that they will receive pure, divine inspiration for the highest good of all.

When the throat chakra is soft, open and free, I know that they will speak with truth, love and compassion.

When we practice psychometry, we rub our hands together and practice feeling and sensing the energy that flows between them, before using this gift to feel and receive downloads of information from an object or item belonging to the person for whom we are giving a reading.

There are also cases when I see unexpected colours in chakras. For example, when I see pink light in the sacral chakra, as well as the customary orange, I know that this is someone who will use their creativity to manifest peace and unconditional love on Earth, as a part of their divine mission. Sometimes, by re-introducing the colour orange to this chakra, the student concerned will become more purposefulness and begin to manifest their creations on Earth in a rich, dynamic and tangible form.

There are often two colours used by the heart chakra. For most people the colour green is most evident in this area, for the purpose of balancing the emotions and creating a healthy emotional environment for harmonious relationships and connections. In the case of those who also display a great deal of pink in this chakra, there is a clear intention to increase, develop and share their understanding of unconditional love - the higher vibration of love. I have often also seen this colour transforming the orange of the sacral chakra into a softer coral colour, among mothers and those who work in fields where unconditional love is a necessity and where the role of mothering and caring for others have caused them to develop this quality over time.

12. Chakra Karma – Healing and Releasing the Past

When we look at a side-view of the energy bodies and chakras, we usually see a succession of trumpet-like structures emanating from the body at each of the chakra points. They trumpet forward from the front of the bodies and backwards from behind. In other words, each of our chakras operates both in front of the body and behind it.

We predominantly use the chakras at the front of the body to absorb, process and interpret new information and learning about the energies around us, while the back chakras often store, process and eventually release the wounds and scars from our past experiences, those which we tend to accumulate on our journey through life. In the case of the chakra at the back of the heart, there is often a huge backlog of unprocessed emotional experiences which becomes lighter when we do the necessary inner work, mostly by forgiving (both ourselves and others) and bringing true wisdom to the way we choose to view these experiences. In this case, forgiveness doesn't mean that we condone the misdeeds of others; it simply means that we decide to put our burdens down and see the experiences from a higher perspective, taking the lessons gained from them and leaving the rest. To forgive others is to make ourselves new every day, and self-forgiveness means that we extend compassion towards ourselves for our earlier mistakes and misdeeds, and no longer berate ourselves for them. When we are able to do this, we grow closer to our original, divine blueprint and increase our ability to become ageless, radiant 5th dimensional beings, wide awake to our eternal selves while living, walking and breathing in a physical body. Welcome to the new Earth!

Of course, being incarnated as a human at this time, I know this may sound like an idealised situation and, essentially, it's one of the things we as human beings tend to struggle with most of our lives. We *can't* always 'just let go' of the past, however hard we try. Forceful emotions tend to stick around for a lot longer than absolutely necessary, and when we feel unheard, misunderstood or experience a lack of compassion from others and a lack of justice in the world, it's sometimes almost impossible to release the thoughts that keep us stuck – thoughts and feelings based in frustration, resentment, loneliness, lack and regret. However, everything we repeatedly think and feel is engraved upon our being and, in the end, these thoughts of frustration and anger only weigh us down, hinder our spiritual and emotional growth and impede our sense of happiness and wellbeing.

Look at the face of someone who knows how to forgive quickly, and you will probably see someone whose youthful complexion belies their true numerical age. There will be a lightness about them, a radiance generated by their determination to live in the moment, unburdened by dark thoughts and ancient shadows. Yes, this will be as apparent in their countenance as a lifetime spent recycling thoughts of revenge, bitterness and malevolence.

Releasing old wounding from the back chakras is one of the most powerful ways of restoring our energy and vitality, and I have worked with many clients whose lives and habitual dark moods have been dramatically transformed as a result of releasing a burdensome energetic past and opening up to a future filled with bright new possibilities.

13. The Importance of Chakra Balancing

We often see the words 'chakra' and 'balancing' together and might wonder what this actually means. We understand that chakra movement and rotation are important for the overall functioning of the energy system. We know that cleansing and clearing are important for maintaining a healthy mind, body and consciousness. We can hazard a guess that the alignment of the seven main chakras – in other words, their even placing in a vertical line, parallel with the spine and extending from the pranic tube – is also important in the mechanical sense. But what impact does this mysterious chakra balancing business have on our day to day reality and our ability to be productive, happy members of society? Through the phenomena I've witnessed in the course of my work, I've come to understand chakra balancing as the even placement, interrelatedness, vertical alignment and similar sizing of the seven main chakras, as they work together to absorb and process energy, light, colour, frequency and experience during our interaction with others and the world around us.

In many cases, we will find that there are some chakras which are much larger or more pronounced than others. For example, in the case of someone who is deeply compassionate or overly emotional, we might see an enlarged heart chakra.

I often see in other light-workers, a diminished and pallid-looking root chakra and an inability to be fully grounded and to function effectively in the material world, and in many of these cases, there is often also an unbalanced enlargement of the upper chakras and a lack of vitality in the lower chakras.

Spiritually focused beings often have issues when it comes to finding satisfactory home conditions, thriving in a regular job and earning and consistent living. They might also have issues in the sacral chakra, as they struggle to manifest their creations onto the physical plane. They might have issues concerning the solar plexus chakra, and constantly feel that they are being controlled or manipulated by others or are endlessly giving their power away to please others.

Conversely, in the case of those who have spent a lifetime focusing on career ambitions and material wealth, there might be an overly enlarged root chakra and in those who have spent a great deal of time focusing on creativity or sexuality, the sacral chakra is often enlarged.

I often see a very healthy and vibrant throat chakra in singers, public speakers or those who chant regularly and, in these cases, this chakra will sometimes set the standard for what we hope to achieve for the other six chakras in order to facilitate a life of holistic fulfilment and balance.

However, size is just a linear description that some will find helpful. Perhaps a more correct approach in chakra balancing is to hold the intention of bringing the chakras to the level of equal and appropriate *functioning* that will be most beneficial in each individual case. So, it's perhaps more appropriate to say that a successful healing session will be focused on creating even levels of dynamism, colour intensity, shape and rotation across all chakras and even, at times, just a simple, intuitive knowing that the system is in balance. Don't worry if you're not a clairvoyant. You can immediately begin to intuit which of your chakras might be out of balance. Simply observe yourself, your life, your habits and behaviours, and as you read through the stories that follow, you might see yourself in some of the protagonists and their experiences. You may also have some new realisations that will help you on your journey towards wholeness.

Spend time each day meditating, and visualising all seven chakras in full colour, rotating and vibrating in perfect harmony in a balanced, healthy and happy way.

14. Energy Clearing and the Chakras

We live in an energetic universe and it's unlikely that a single day will ever go by when you will be completely free of external energies. We are constantly engaging with the energies of other individuals and with the collective energy that flows from every thought that is sent out into the collective field. If you are an empath, you already know all about these energy exchanges and the way that certain people, places or circumstances will drain, deplete of depress your energy field when you come into contact with them, or interact with them, even for a short time. When it comes to keeping our energy clear and in balance, we cannot overlook the effect of these external energies. We are living in incredible times of collective transformation and personal sensitivity to vibrational shifts and changes.

If you are here because you are at the beginning of your journey of spiritual awakening, it might have been a powerful and confusing energetic or psychic encounter that led you to this book. You might be trying to find answers to questions about why you feel so exhausted when you spend time with certain people, why you were able to feel stabbing pains when standing close to the unpleasant energy of a bully who recently made your life miserable, or how on earth it could be possible to become anxious, withdrawn and despondent after spending time with someone who is habitually depressive and cynical.

You might have spent many years wondering why you feel virtually disabled when you spend time with certain family members or why your boss's face is the last thing you see as you attempt to drift off to sleep at night. You might be wondering why your dreams are violent, weird or just plain unsettling whenever you sleep in certain people's homes or why you also find yourself hunched over, in an unconscious attempt to protect your solar plexus when a certain colleague enters the room. You might have found yourself developing mysterious headaches in certain company or frequent bouts of confusion - constantly changing your mind about the path you wish to take in life after spending time in the company of yet another forceful and opinionated friend, partner or family member.

In almost every case of psychic entanglement I have worked on with clients and students, the chords and attachments sent by others are attached to one or more of the chakras. In some cases, the psychic invasion was so intense that the person under attack was unable think for themselves and had lost the ability to feel and know their own desires and intentions, until these chords and attachments were released and dissolved. I have seen many cases where the throat chakra was in pain because someone the client was connected to was desperate to speak to them or was waiting – with a great deal of anxiety and attachment - for the answer to a question, or for a call to be returned.

I have seen clients who were consistently unable to become independent and autonomous in the world until chords attaching them to a controlling parent were dissolved from the root chakra.

Of course there are also many cases where toxic energy sent by an immature soul has manifested as a generically oppressive overshadowing in the wider energy-field of the student or client in question, but I've very rarely found it possible to work on a complete energy-clearing without paying some attention to releasing stagnant energy from specific chakras.

So, by now, you'll be much clearer about the importance of the chakras and the role they play in our psychic, emotional, mental and even physical health and wellbeing.

In the following chapters, I'm going to demonstrate, using scenes from the lives of seven fictional characters, how an under-functioning or dysfunctional chakra might look, feel and be experienced as a set of life conditions, circumstances, tendencies and experiences.

At the end of each of these stories, I'll also share meditations, healing recommendations and ideas about the changes one might expect to see as a result of healing. Please keep in mind that these stories are simply a guide to enable us to focus on the chakras one by one. It's important to remember that none of the chakras exist in isolation, and it's unusual to find only one blocked chakra in an individual. I encourage you to take a holistic view and to see the chakras as a continuum, a series of interrelated organisms all working together to create harmony and balance.

If you do recognise your own experience in any of these stories, I hope you will find the related healing tips useful. If you experience a powerful realisation at any point, please feel free to stop reading and meditate on what you're learning. I hope this book works well as an interactive healing tool, and that you'll also enjoy using the tables I have provided, as a series of quick guides to assist you on your chakra healing journey.

15. Finding Your Feet: Balancing the Root Chakra

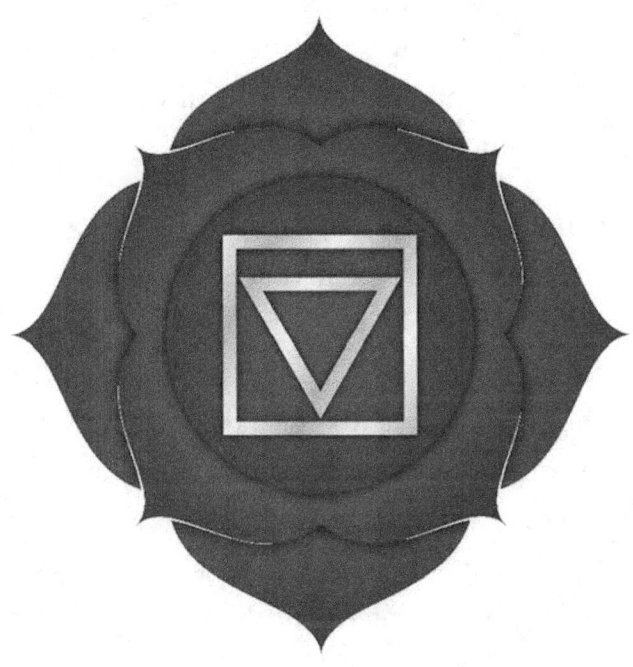

John was a talented man and a gifted artist. He was utterly devoted to his art work and would spend hour after hour perfecting his technique and his understanding of colour, shape, form and texture. He had a sharp eye for things no one else could see, both in the natural world and in the people, places and objects around him. Even as a child, John had shown great promise as an artist, and at school his work had always been chosen for displays and special school assemblies.

John had been a quiet but popular child at school. He was friendly, kind and compassionate towards his classmates, even though he was incredibly shy and at times, even a little withdrawn. He found it difficult to speak to new people and often sat at the back of the class, doodling or painting pictures in his mind while the teacher addressed rest of the class. He was often described as a daydreamer and was known for bumping into things and tripping over his feet. There were days when he seemed calm and contented in class and other days when he seemed nervous and unsettled.

John grew up in an abusive household. His father was an alcoholic and his mother spent the entirety of their marriage tiptoeing around him, ensuring that his frequent angry flare-ups were kept to a minimum for the sake of the children. As he grew older, John began to realise that his family wasn't like everyone else's. He never felt truly safe at home and he longed to be free of a home life that was fraught with difficulties and lack. There were often arguments at home, mostly about money, and John was often caught in the middle of them. As the eldest of four children, he felt responsible for everyone but completely impotent at the same time. He was just a kid, what could he possibly do that would make a difference!

John made a habit of retreating into his artwork, his special world, and even though he often fought with his siblings over pencils, paper and basic school supplies, he would always find away to draw and paint. He felt safe and secure, as long as he could make markings on paper. It was his way of creating a world where everything was always perfect and beautiful.

When John was eleven, his mother left his father and took him and his siblings to live with his step father, who was also equally abusive. He wasn't violent towards John and his siblings but when his mother would go out to work, John felt uncomfortable about the strange things he would ask of him. He knew in his heart that they were wrong, but his stepfather would often threaten him if he so much as mentioned sharing these secrets with his mother.

Every evening when his mother went out to work, John's stepfather would reinforce his warning and threaten John with future violence. So, John kept quiet. His mother finally seemed happy. She was financially independent and was a hard worker who was frequently rewarded and promoted.

Despite his deep-rooted fear of his stepfather, one day, when John had become completely and utterly despondent, he asked his mother why she had to go out to work all the time. His already exhausted mother flew into a rage and asked him who he thought was going to earn money and put food on the table if she didn't. Crushed, hopeless, helpless and trapped, John retreated to his room to paint his special, magical world and dream of the day when he would be able to escape.

When that day finally came and John left home to go to art college, he was overwhelmed with guilt about leaving his siblings behind and utterly distraught about the sort of life they might have to endure in his absence, but he was free now and he needed time and space to heal from the past and make something of his life so he could one day return to help them.

As he relaxed into his university studies, John was immediately recognised for every piece of work he submitted, but he still had a habit of bumping into things and often seemed spaced out and incommunicative. He was unwilling to make eye contact and would often retreat into himself, preferring to study and paint in the evenings, rather than joining his new friends for drinks and socialising. He hated alcohol, hated what it did to people and couldn't stand to hear the way people would talk about being famous and getting rich, as if money was all they were really interested in. All he wanted to do make the world a better place. He saw money as corrupt and toxic, and even despised himself for needing it for his survival.

John never saw himself as someone who was hiding away from the world; he saw himself as a true artist and, after all, wasn't that what true artists did!? – they suffered for their art, eschewing all the trinkets and baubles that were dangled temptingly in front of them, in favour of an opportunity to create a better, brighter world.

Most of the time, John felt disconnected from the material world and yet he was also desperately worried about the future. To his friends, he seemed withdrawn and unfathomable. However, he effortlessly gained a first for his degree, and it was unanimously agreed that he was a promising young artist, but he somehow just didn't feel connected to his success. There were many days when he wasn't sure he felt anything. His friends would often joke that he was like a being from another planet. His hands were always cold, even in the most scorching summer temperatures and he had an air of someone who was always walking on tiptoes. He would tire easily and often had a sense of hopelessness and distraction that only went away when he was painting, discussing art or watching art documentaries.

After college, John was offered a full scholarship to complete an MA program, but he was tired of studying and wanted to find his own way in the world and prove that he could make something of himself.

He found a job working for a graphic design company and within a few months was promoted to team leader. He felt uncomfortable telling people what to do but it was his job and he needed the money.

He moved out of student accommodation and rented a flat a few minutes away from work, but within a year he was told that the company was closing and there would only be a small redundancy package which could only be offered to staff who had been working with the company for more than a year. John had just reached his eleventh month working for the company and the rules were rigid.

Determined not to be beaten, he decided to set up in business on his own but somehow, despite his earlier success and his impeccable reputation, he always seemed to be either struggling to get clients or struggling to keep them. Whenever he did manage to acquire and keep several clients at once, he would almost immediately notice something major going wrong with his car or that a large household appliance suddenly needed to be replaced, always keeping him at the same level of economic deficit. It was almost as if he'd been programmed never to live comfortably.

When a distant relative died and left him a reasonably large sum of money, John finally gave himself a break. He was tired of working twenty-four hours a day, seven days a week. He had to think of his long-term future. So, he invested money in some stocks and shares (two weeks before they took an unmitigated dip) and treated himself to a specialist art summer school with one of his all-time idols in the modern art world.

It was on this trip that he met Carol and began a life-changing intimate relationship. He shared everything with her: his thoughts about art, his painful upbringing and his previous struggles with money, his recent inheritance, and his fears about the future. Carol was such a great listener and they had so much in common. It was like coming home. In fact, after just a few months of dating, John realised he wanted to share his home with Carol. Business was booming, as a result of the money he had been able to invest into advertising, and it seemed as if John's life had been transformed. He was overjoyed to be painting again and had toyed with the idea of putting on his first show or even going back to college to complete his MA.

For the first few months of living with Carol, John felt as if he had finally found the happiness he'd been denied his whole life. He was still bumping into things, but he was even able to laugh at himself now, and to his relief, Carol would laugh right along with him... until, of course, the first time he noticed that she actually seemed to be laughing *at* him... just slightly at first... but definitely ... yes, he was sure of it. There was no mistaking that sudden change in tone.

Of course, it was very subtle at first, but John recognised the feeling immediately from his childhood - the feeling of being sneered at for not being quite good enough. The feeling of questioning himself and telling himself he was imagining things. In fact, the first time it happened, he put it down to his over-sensitivity, but when he noticed it happening more frequently, he felt a sick feeling in the pit of his stomach. The first time Carol screamed at him and called him a f__ing idiot, he spent several days in bed recovering from the extreme psychic attack and trying desperately to regain his lost sense of idealisation.

Of course, Carol apologised profusely and explained calmly that she'd recently been under a lot of pressure at work and that she would try not to let her emotions get the better of her in future.

John forgave her tantrums and spent the next two weeks making up for lost time with valuable clients and winning them back after missing a few deadlines, and for a while, things went back to normal. The wonderful woman he had met at the retreat was back, and, so, he carefully put the episode out of his mind.

It took a while for him to notice that whenever they went out together, Carol would order whisky and rum and would inevitably keep drinking until she was fell asleep. It took a while for him to realise that the aggressive shouting episodes, followed by ardent apologies and make-up sessions, were becoming more frequent, and it took years for him to finally realise that he was struggling financially once again and was feeling fundamentally unhappy, unsafe and impoverished in every way.

Eventually, when life became unbearable, he moved in with an old college friend and found himself a job cleaning in a restaurant, to make some quick, easy money. Reassured when an online graphic design customer added a large tip via the donation button on his website, John saw this as a small sign that maybe his fortunes were finally improving, and he was sending good energy out into the universe once again. He was later disappointed when the same person invited him to contribute to a fundraiser just a few weeks later. Conflicted about what to do, John gave back two thirds of the original donation to contribute to the fundraiser…. and still felt guilty… and generally unsafe…He constantly worried about money and lived in fear of never having enough to cover his bills or feed himself. Problems with lower back pain made it difficult for him to cope with the long shifts he needed to do at the restaurant, simply in order to survive. However, with the relationship with Carol now far behind him, he was free to make new choices that would move his life forward in a more favourable direction. His friends were relieved to see him trying to get back on his feet again, but no one could really understand why he wasn't applying for a good job in graphic design, or reapplying for that scholarship…

With a healed root chakra, John would gradually learn to trust life again. He would no longer attract situations or connections that reinforced his feelings of being unsafe in the world, and if he did, he would trust himself enough to deal with them confidently and securely. He would gradually notice that he was worrying less about money and, as a result, would begin to see more opportunities to improve his finances and his general feeling of safety and security in the world. He would begin to believe that he was deserving of good things. He would feel more grounded and have fewer panic attacks about his finances, and it's more than likely that his lower back pain would gradually decrease and possibly disappear altogether. If he allowed himself to heal, he would begin to feel generally more at home in the world and more ready to enjoy of all forms of abundance. He would begin to feel as if the earth was a safe and loving home. Ultimately, effective healing would enable him to release his childhood wounds, build a firm foundation in life and move on to a brighter future.

15.1 Healing and Maintenance of the Root chakra

So how do you know if your root chakra is out of balance? If you answer yes to three or more of the questions below, it's highly likely that it is.

1. Do you often feel spaced out and find it difficult to get grounded?

2. Do you struggle to make ends meet financially, despite working very hard and frequently receiving lucky breaks?

3. Do you often feel generally unsafe in the world?

4. Did you experience childhood trauma that made you want to escape from the world, either literally or by using your imagination?

5. Do you regularly suffer from lower back pain but have no physical reason, injury or condition that explains it?

If your root chakra is blocked, out of balance or in need of healing, try some of the remedies and practices below to help bring it back into balance and restore harmony and wellbeing.

Meditation for Healing the Root Chakra

Close your eyes and sit in a comfortable position with your feet planted firmly on the floor.

Breathe deeply and visualise white light streaming down from above and creating a thick, protective energy bubble around you.

Place your hands on the base of your spine or anywhere in the root chakra area that feels right for you.

Visualise deep ruby red light streaming down into the root chakra from your hands.

If you have trouble visualising, simply close your eyes and repeat the following words:

Rich, ruby red light, rich, ruby red light. Continue repeating these words mentally and silently, until you're able to believe in, and possibly even see glimpses or flashes of this deep, ruby red light streaming into your root chakra, healing, enriching and cleansing it with an influx of its true colour vibration.

Carry out this meditation for approximately twenty minutes or until you feel peaceful, recharged and re-energised. Making a regular habit of working on each of your chakras in this way, using the uniquely appropriate chakra colours, will ensure that all your chakras are effectively charged, energised and in perfect balance with each other.

Future Care and Maintenance of the Root Chakra

As much as time allows, be sure to use this meditation to regularly recharge, heal and balance your root chakra, but in order keep this chakra whole and healthy and your outlook positive and bright, here are some other measures you can take to ensure the ongoing health of this chakra.

Healing Behaviours for Maintaining Good Root Chakra Health

If you've spent several years or even decades with a depleted or unbalanced root chakra, it might take some time for you to restore it to full vitality but rest assured that you can do it with patience and with regular use of these tips and techniques.

Spend time getting to know yourself as a physical being. What are the things you love most about the physical experience on life on Earth? The smell of wet earth, warm, luxurious showers with creamy, naturally scented soap, massages with essential oils, chocolates and perfume? Rose petals in your bath? Tree hugging and walks in the forest, feeling the sun or the wind on your skin? Dancing with a lover? Curry and rice? Raw food concoctions or roasted root vegetables?

Think of something you can do regularly to enhance your appreciation of your physical body and all the scrummy things that only life in the material realm can offer. Spend more time walking outdoors with your feet on the grass and the earth rather than on concrete. Hug more, kiss more, smile more.

Using Colour to Heal and Recharge the Root Chakra

Wear more rich, ruby red tones and try to avoid getting stuck in a pattern of wearing dark colours simply to avoid drawing attention to yourself. Use more earthy, autumnal tones in your clothing and furnishings, and bring more of these into your daily life to increase your awareness of them and allow your mind and your energy-field to absorb their benefits as you go about your daily routines.

Crystals for Root Chakra Cleansing and Balancing

Lie down in a quiet room and place cleansed and energised pieces of red jasper, red carnelian, bloodstone or garnet crystals on your root chakra area for twenty minutes or so. Try this once a week until you get used to the feeling of these powerful energies. While you're healing this chakra, you can also carry these stones around with you or wear them on a necklace or bracelet.

Essential Oils for Clearing and Healing the Root Chakra

Massage your root chakra area with powerful, rich, deep, earthy fragranced oils such as: Cedarwood, Benzoin, Patchouli and Black Pepper. Please remember to always dilute your essential oils with a good quality carrier oil before applying them to the skin, and make sure there are no contraindications to your use of essential oils.

Yoga for Clearing and Healing the Root Chakra

If you're a yoga practitioner and have no impediments to physical exercise, you might like to try the following yoga poses to help open, clear, balance and release energy toxic energy from the root chakra:

- **Spinal flexing exercises, e.g. cat pose**

- **Head to knee, forward bend pose**

- **Wide-legged forward bend pose**

- **Locust or half locust pose**

- **Knee to chest pose**

Remember that it's always best to study yoga with a qualified instructor, and if you're studying at home, please be gentle with yourself and go at a slow and steady pace that you know you can handle. Sometimes we gain the best results from the smallest of movements carried out in just the right way.

See the healing table at the end of this book for a comprehensive cheat sheet on all the tips and techniques that will help you to strengthen this chakra.

Happy root chakra healing!

16. Uncomfortably Numb: Balancing the Sacral Chakra

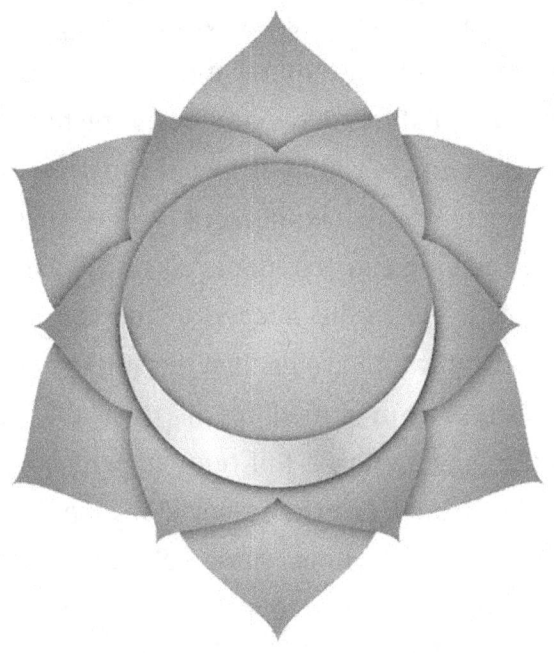

Deborah couldn't remember a time when she had ever felt genuinely happy. On the surface, she seemed to have everything: a loving partner, two amazing children (despite years of gynaecological issues and problems conceiving), a wonderful circle of supportive friends, a great job and a wonderful, warm and loving home. Yet she still felt numb and generally depressed. She would often get angry with herself for even daring to feel this way when she had so much to be thankful for. How could she even dare to be miserable when there were people starving in the world, and people who didn't even have a comfortable bed to sleep in at night?! She would torture herself with these thoughts in her darkest moments but, somehow, she still felt numb, and however great her life looked from the outside, on the inside she felt as if there was something missing.

Deborah was often told she had everything going for her, but she felt sluggish, indifferent, unfulfilled and emotionally constipated. Her libido was at an all time low and her punishing work hours, coupled with the endless round of school runs, meal preparation, babysitting arrangements, homework supervision and school events, left her feeling exhausted, out of control and even more disappointed in herself. She needed a holiday, but there was nowhere she really wanted to go. Just getting through a day was enough, and she was horrified to discover that her greatest pleasure in life was having a full hour in which to completely numb out in front of the television before collapsing emotionlessly into bed, in a miserable, self-loathing heap.

Sometimes when she was baking cakes with the children at weekends, she would fantasise about being a TV chef or having a Youtube channel and spending all her time baking and making yummy, fun things. Then she'd snap back into the real world, where another overwhelming collection of work emails was patiently waiting for her attention.

On the rare occasions when she went out shopping for clothes with a friend, she would daydream about being a personal shopper. At the make-up counter, she would dream of being a make-artist or a beautician. Perhaps she wasn't so happy with her job after all.. In the evenings she'd be snappy and irritable, and in the morning, she would wake up feeling nervous about the future for no particular reason.

If Deborah learned how to heal and balance her sacral chakra, she would gradually begin to feel calmer, and more in control of her life. She would create more time and space to explore her creativity, and to reconnect with her feelings and her sensual, feminine side. She would begin to see these things as important and find ways to include them in her life. She would speak up about feeling overwhelmed and enlist more help. Her feelings of low self-esteem would begin to dissolve, allowing her to accept help without feeling as if she was somehow to blame for not being able to cope with an insane workload. Gradually, as her workload decreased, she would find peace and balance returning, and her feelings of numbness would begin to dissipate. Over time, her life would begin to feel less like a rollercoaster ride, and she would gradually begin to feel a powerful reconnection with her creativity and spontaneity. Her sense of humour would return and her panic about life would subside, allowing her to give herself occasional treats and spend more time doing fun things. In time, she might even learn to smile inwardly and to feel deep gratitude and appreciation for her life, without guilt or shame.

16.1 Healing and Maintenance of the Sacral Chakra

How do you know if your sacral chakra is out of balance? If you answer yes to three or more of the questions below, it's highly likely that it is.

- Do you often feel bored, listless and generally disconnected from your life?

- Do you often feel numb, apathetic and disinterested in life and/or work and secretly dream of doing something creative?

- Have you lost faith in your creative abilities and/or your ability to create a better life?

- Do you often feel out of control and overwhelmed?

- Do you feel your sexuality is completely out of balance, causing you to either obsess about sex or feel a complete lack of interest?

If your sacral chakra is blocked, out of balance or in need of healing, try some of the remedies and practices below to help bring it back into balance and restore harmony and wellbeing.

Meditation for Healing the Sacral Chakra

Close your eyes and sit in a comfortable position with your feet planted firmly on the floor.

Breathe deeply and visualise white light streaming down from above and creating a thick, protective energy bubble around you.

Place your hands on your lower abdomen and breathe deeply into this area.

Visualise a rich, deep orange light streaming down into the sacral chakra, through your hands.

If you have trouble visualising, simply close your eyes and repeat the following words:

Rich, deep, orange light, rich, deep, orange light. Continue repeating these words mentally and silently, until you're able to believe in, and possibly even see glimpses or flashes of this deep, orange light streaming into your sacral chakra, healing, enriching and cleansing this chakra its true colour vibration.

Carry out this meditation for approximately twenty minutes or until you feel peaceful, recharged and re-energised. Making a regular habit of working on each of your chakras in this way, using the uniquely appropriate chakra colours, will ensure that all your chakras are recharged, re-energised and in perfect balance with each other.

Future Care and Maintenance of the Sacral Chakra

As much as time allows, be sure to use this meditation to regularly recharge, heal and balance your sacral chakra, but in order keep this chakra whole and healthy and your outlook positive and bright, here are some measures you can take to ensure the ongoing health of this chakra.

Healing Behaviours for Maintaining Good Sacral Chakra Health

Indulge your creativity by taking up a creative hobby. Even if you don't consider yourself to be particularly creative, there is sure to be something you can create. For example, create a sumptuous meal, bake a dreamy cake, start a daily journal, explore creative home décor, make your own greetings cards, start a board games night, join a beginners dance class, knit a scarf, create and frame a photo montage of your dearest friends, family members and memories. Get creative in your thinking and come up with some new ideas of your own.

If you've been denying yourself a lapsed creative passion you once had, reawaken your interest in this area and your passion will surely awaken in other areas too! Be honest with yourself about what you might need to change in order to bring the fun and spontaneity back into your life.

If you feel overwhelmed, ask for help. If you feel generally unimpressed with life, try to reduce or eliminate the use of artificial stimulants, such as caffeine, and dig deep into the untapped well of dynamic, pranic energy that's just waiting to energise your chakras, your energy field and ultimately, your life.

Using Colour to Heal and Recharge the Sacral Chakra

Wear more orange and golden tones, and generally create more interest and excitement in your style of dress. Get creative with scarves, shawls, neckties, trendy waistcoats, accessories, hair colouring and uniquely decorative fashion items that allow you to express your true inner character and your naturally creative soul. If you feel unappreciated or unseen, try to love and appreciate yourself more by dressing well and giving yourself little treats that make you feel special and cared for.

Use more orange in your home furnishings and bring more of these cheerful tones into your life, to increase your awareness of them and allow your mind and your energy-field to absorb their cheerful vibration and the uplifting and life-affirming feelings they bring, as you go about your daily routines.

Crystals for Sacral Chakra Cleansing and Balancing

Lie down in a quiet room and place a few cleansed and energised pieces of orange carnelian, citrine or tiger's eye crystals on your lower abdomen for twenty minutes or so. Try this once a week until you get used to the feeling of these powerful energies. While you're healing this chakra, you can also carry these stones around with you, or wear them on a necklace or bracelet.

Essential Oils for Clearing and Healing the Sacral Chakra

Gently massage your lower abdomen with orange, sweet orange, neroli, ginger or cinnamon oil. Please remember to always dilute your essential oils with a good quality carrier oil before applying them directly to the body and do some research to make sure there are no contraindications to your use of essential oils.

Yoga for Clearing and Healing the Sacral Chakra

If you're a yoga practitioner and have no impediments to physical exercise, you might like to try the following yoga poses to help open, clear and release toxic energy from the sacral chakra:

- **Full boat pose**

- **Cobra pose**

- **Bound angle pose**

- **Pelvic rock, tilt and rotation exercises**

Remember that it's always best to study yoga with a qualified instructor, and if you're studying at home, please be gentle with yourself and go at a slow and steady pace that you know you can manage. Sometimes we gain the best results from the smallest of movements carried out in just the right way.

See the healing table at the end of this book for a comprehensive cheat sheet on all the tips and techniques that will help you to strengthen this chakra.

Happy sacral chakra healing!

17. Drawing a Line in the Sand: Balancing the Solar Plexus Chakra

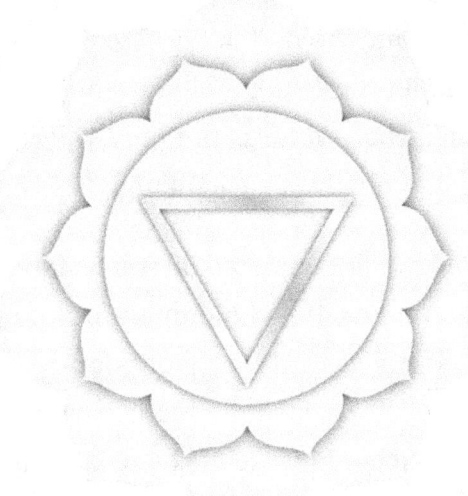

Melanie prided herself on being a kind and compassionate person. There was nothing she wouldn't do to help a friend in need. She'd been that way for as long as she could remember, in fact, it wasn't something she had ever really thought about that much; it was just who he was. Friends knew they could call her at any time of day or night, and she would gladly listen to their worries and woes until they felt better.

Melanie's husband was exasperated with her. He couldn't understand why she wouldn't just say no! There were many times when he would awaken in the middle of the night to the sound of mumbling, only to hear his wife consoling yet another friend who was stressed out about work, worried about her relationship or just generally in need of a sympathetic ear.

Melanie found it incredibly difficult to say no because she was an empath. Not only did she sympathise with the sadness and misfortunes of others, she could also feel them. So, if a friend was in pain and needed her help, she would feel obliged to give it. She would have no choice but to listen for as long as they needed her to and let them talk it all out until they felt better. It sometimes seemed that this was the only way that she, herself could feel better and finally get a good night's sleep.

Melanie nearly always felt depleted after speaking to her friends. There was no one in her life who didn't absolutely exhaust her. But what could she do!? It didn't feel good to just turn them away! So, instead, she turned to food, partly as a source of comfort and perhaps, unconsciously,to develop some extra padding, to protect herself from the psychic and energetic intrusion. Of course, she hadn't *wanted* to start gaining weight, but Melanie was swimming in vampire soup and needed something to help her to stay afloat.

She didn't notice her comfort eating getting out of hand. At first it was just an extra helping of dessert here, a reassuring bar of chocolate there and a general lack of energy everywhere. There was no inclination or energy left for exercising after a long, hard day of listening to, consoling and pleasing everyone. She didn't even notice the weight piling on at first; it was just a slight tightening of the waistband here, a seemingly shrunken sweater there, but somehow, she suddenly couldn't stop eating. She just didn't want to. Somehow excessive eating felt a lot easier than saying no.

Every week she would begin her new, healthy regime on Monday mornings, vowing that she wouldn't have any sweets or cakes that week, but by the time she had endured another two hours of her best friend dumping a lifetime of woes into her solar plexus, she was ready to have chocolate pumped into her bloodstream via intravenous drip. When she began keeping extra packets of family sized chocolate buttons under the bed, to quickly replace lost energy after chatting with friends, she knew there was a problem, but she reasoned that even when she had been a healthier eater, she had always found it impossible to lose weight, especially around the tummy area.

Melanie's mother had a habit of sucking all the joy and vitality out of her life, and after her visits Melanie would feel as if her innards had been scooped out with a large wooden ladle, and on top of being utterly depleted, she would also feel nervous, and anxious that she hadn't done enough to make her mother's visit enjoyable, or that she just generally wasn't good enough in some other, mysterious way that she just hadn't managed to figure out yet.

Melanie began to develop digestive issues and to have frequent problems with gas and nausea. She often felt as if she'd been kicked in the stomach and would sit with her shoulders hunched over, to protect her solar plexus. At night, she would always need a hot water bottle on her stomach, sometimes even in summer. It made her feel comforted. Her husband begged her to start setting appropriate boundaries so that she could at least get a decent night's sleep, but her entire means of gaining self-worth had become built around being able to please people and make them feel better. She needed to feel needed, and the angrier she felt about her weight gain, the more she needed the external validation of being needed, to bolster up her crumbling self-esteem.

If Melanie chose to work on strengthening her solar plexus chakra and building a protective shield around this delicate psychic centre, she would gradually begin to feel safe again without using food as a defence mechanism. Over time, she would feel stronger within herself and gain more clarity about how to protect and shield her energy field and her chakras from the vampiric chords and attachments that were making her life a sleepless nightmare. In this way, she would finally begin to put an end to the controlling and manipulative behaviours of her friends and family. As her solar plexus became stronger, she would feel less of the push and pull of other people's energies and would feel free to experiment with appropriate dietary choices, extreme self-care and strong boundaries, sharing compassion from a position of love and choice rather than from anxiety and obligation.

If you suffer with similar issues, it's important to remember that being an empath makes you a beautiful person - exactly the kind of person the world currently needs - but an inability to take care of yourself will leave you too vulnerable to toxic people, situations and addictions to be truly effective in the world, and those who prey upon this vulnerability will just keep on taking if you let them.

The solar plexus is one of the most powerful centres of psychic perception, and yet it can be the most vulnerable of all the chakras, the soft underbelly, so to speak. Learning how to take care of this psychic gateway can mean the difference between being an enlightened and empowered empath and a boundary-less and disempowered psychic sponge.

17.1 Healing and Maintenance of the Solar Plexus Chakra

So how do you know if your solar plexus chakra is out of balance? If you answer yes to three or more of the questions below, it's highly likely that it is.

1. Are you a people pleaser - do you often say yes when you really want to say no?

2. Do you consider yourself to be an empath – in other words, do you frequently feel the pain of others?

3. Were you ever made to feel disempowered by an overbearing parent or sibling?

4. Were you ever told you were terrible at making good choices and decisions, and do you now have trouble trusting your own judgement as a result?

5. Are you a comfort eater who eats as a way of dealing with anxiety – do you have trouble losing weight even when you eat a healthy diet?

If your solar plexus chakra is depleted, blocked, out of balance or in need of healing, try some of the remedies and practices below to help bring it back into balance and restore harmony and wellbeing.

Meditation for Healing the Solar Plexus Chakra

Close your eyes and sit in a comfortable position with your feet planted firmly on the floor.

Breathe deeply and visualise white light streaming down from above and creating a thick, protective energy bubble around you.

Place your hands on your solar plexus and breathe deeply into this area.

Visualise rich, golden light and pure, sunshine yellow light streaming down into this chakra from your hands.

If you have trouble visualising, simply close your eyes and repeat the following words:

Yellow light, golden light, rich, deep golden light. Yellow light, golden light, rich, deep golden light. Continue repeating these words mentally and silently, until you're able to believe in, and possibly even see, glimpses or flashes of these yellow and golden lights streaming into your solar plexus chakra, healing, enriching and cleansing it with its true colour vibration.

Carry out this meditation for approximately thirty minutes, or until you feel strong, protected peaceful, recharged and re-energised.

Making a regular habit of working on each of your chakras in this way, using the uniquely appropriate chakra colours, will ensure that all your chakras remain clear, energised and in perfect balance with each other.

Future Care and Maintenance of the Solar Plexus Chakra

As much as time allows, be sure to use this meditation regularly, to heal and balance your solar plexus chakra, but in order keep this chakra whole and healthy and your outlook positive and bright, here are some other measures you can take to ensure the ongoing health of the solar plexus chakra.

Healing Behaviours for Maintaining Optimal Solar Plexus Chakra Health

As much as possible, stay away from negative people and minimise contact with those who drain your vital energy. Notice how your stomach and solar plexus feel when you spend time with certain people. People who are chronically depressed or those who are constantly complaining of various injuries and mysterious illnesses are notoriously vampiric in nature. Of course, we all get down from time to time, and anyone can occasionally lose their way or go through a rough period. Try not to become an energy snob and allow an obsession with guarding your chakras at all costs rob you of your compassion. However, if you have a long-term history of feeling utterly depleted and dispirited immediately after spending time with a certain individual, and if just five minutes in their company has you dreaming about lying on the pavement inhaling an entire sweetshop, after weeks of healthy eating, clearly something has gone wrong!

This delicate psychic centre, also known as the psychic brain, seems to be a special little sweet spot for energy vampires. Although (in most cases) much of their vampirism is entirely unconscious, these hungry little bunnies will suck your energy out through a giant straw and leave you gasping for breath without remorse. Please take note and vow to stop giving your power away.

Stay away from guilt trips of any kind. If the energy vampire is a parent or other family member who also happens to be supporting you financially, work hard to gain your independence and pay your way equally in all social and living situations so that you won't feel obliged to give back in the form of a huge dollop of time and energy. These things can be very difficult to measure and are seldom acknowledged and appreciated enough to be logged as a fair exchange offering – your vampire will simply become a bottomless pit and your life will somehow, mysteriously, never seem to move forward.

We all have equal access to the same divine energy source. Your time and your lifeforce are some of the precious gifts of your sovereign state of being, here on Earth. Do not squander them like an insignificant afterthought. Share them wisely and generously with those who give back to you, or those who recognise and value these gifts enough to ask nicely for them and agree to receive them within a structured time and context – for example in a pre-arrange Reiki session.

Have sleepovers only in places that feel comfortable and safe to you and refuse to let yourself be sleep-robbed by night-time prana thieves and their roaming tentacles.

If you are extra sensitive to being drained from this psychic power centre, spend time meditating on how to become quietly and lovingly assertive in ways that suit your nature. Develop strong boundaries and learn to say no, kindly.

Most of all, learn that it's important to be kind to yourself. A little trick I used to use was to ask myself the following question: If the roles were reversed and I was the other person in this situation, is this how I would be behaving? If you are appalled at the very idea, imagine for a second how you *would* behave in a similar situation. For most empaths, the answer might be: *well, if I was in that much pain, I would probably spend some quiet time healing and recharging my energies until I felt much better, and then if I really felt the need to talk this over with a friend, I would first ask them if this was a good time to talk. If they said it wasn't, I would hear this the first time and return to my self-healing, journaling, meditation, chanting, singing, dancing in the rain or any other activity from the vast range of wonderful things I do to make myself feel better.*

So why don't you deserve the same courtesy?

Mentally switching roles in this way has been one of the most life-changing methods I've used for identifying poor behaviour. As a natural empath, I want everyone to feel good, so I don't always see (or feel) bad behaviour coming. Be kind to yourself. Be your own best friend, the one who truly values your kindness and sweetness and who will be there in your corner, through thick and thin.

As a sensitive soul on a dynamic and conscious quest to gain spiritual understanding, you may find that your light often attracts unconscious people who are not necessarily on the same path, or who claim to be on the same path but are not necessarily doing the same depth of work. They may not have spent decades honing their ability to connect with a higher power. It's entirely possible that they're not currently spending hours, days weeks, months or even a lifetime on energy-clearing and vibration-raising techniques. They might not know or care about increasing their awareness so that they can become infinitely recharged, inspired, uplifted and full of vitality. Gently guide them back towards the infinite light and try not to be seduced by anyone who says: *Oh, wow, I always feel so much better after spending time with you!* Before getting carried away by flattery, notice how *you* feel after the encounter. Is it working for you too? If you arrived at their home full of the joys of spring and within an hour of listening to their latest catalogue of disasters, you feel tempted to ask if there's anywhere you could go to have a quick nap before going home, you might want to revaluate that connection.

Be strong, be patient but above all, be kind to yourself. Keep on keeping on. You will find your tribe one day. Your tribe is already looking for you. If the person you're trying to help is a bottomless pit that can't ever be filled but who doggedly refuses to ever feel better, even momentarily, and if they continue to regale you with endless complaints of slights, injuries and mysteriously undiagnosed bodily malfunctions, they're not there for solutions, they're there for energy. Develop a habit of lovingly guiding them to the same practices and resources you have used to create wholeness within yourself..and wish them the very best of luck trying them all out!

Using Colour to Heal and Recharge the Solar Plexus Chakra

Wear more yellow and golden tones and opt for gold or gold-coloured jewellery instead of silver. Buy yourself some sunflowers and have sunflower pictures and summertime-themed prints on your walls. Use these colours in your clothing and furnishings and bring more of these golden tones into your life to increase your awareness of them and allow your mind and your energy-field to absorb their uplifting benefits as you go about your daily routines.

Crystals for Solar Plexus Chakra Cleansing and Balancing

Lie down in a quiet room and place a few cleansed and nicely charged pieces of citrine, amber or tiger's eye crystals on your solar plexus area for twenty minutes or so. Try this once a week until you get used to the feel of these powerful energies. While you're healing this chakra, you can also carry these stones around with you or wear them on a necklace or bracelet.

Essential Oils for Clearing and Healing the Sacral Chakra

Massage your stomach and solar plexus with grapefruit, clary sage, lemon, lemongrass, fennel and/or peppermint essential oil.

Please remember to always dilute your essential oils with a good quality carrier oil before applying them directly to the body.

Yoga for Clearing and Healing the Solar Plexus Chakra

If you're a yoga practitioner and have no impediments to physical exercise, you might like to try the following yoga poses to help open, clear and release in that area:

- Bow pose

- Fish pose

- Half lord of the fishes pose, and other twisting poses (use your clairsentience here, and learn to feel the energy moving in this centre. This will be of great benefit to you in choosing the correct poses and for discerning when you need to clear or shield this chakra).

- Salute to the sun

Remember that it's always best to study yoga with a qualified instructor, and if you're studying at home, please be gentle with yourself and go at a slow and steady pace that you know you can handle. Sometimes we gain the best results from the smallest of movements carried out in just the right way. See the healing table at the end of this book for a comprehensive cheat sheet on all the tips and techniques that will help you to strengthen each chakra. Happy solar plexus chakra healing!

18. Dances with the Lone Wolf: Balancing the Heart Chakra

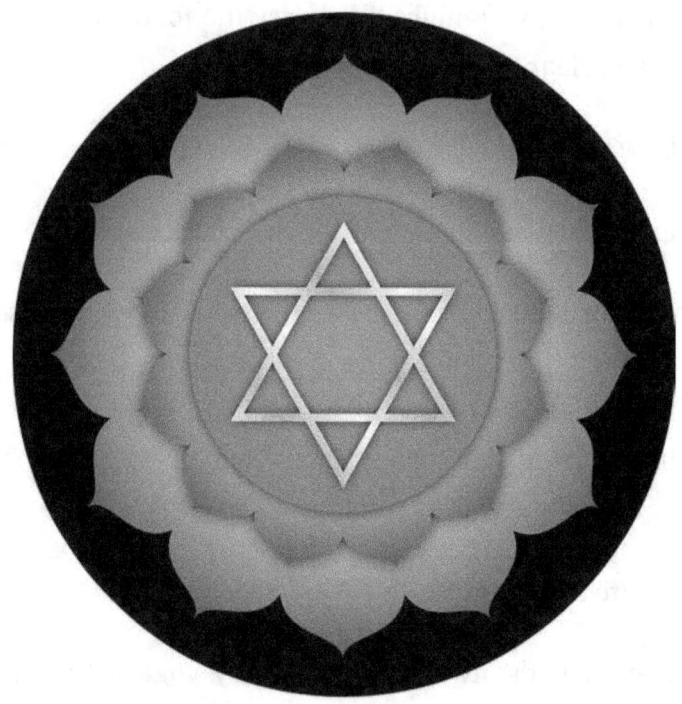

Jack was a loner. He liked being alone. At least, that's what he would tell himself, and anyone else who would ask. His friends were always so full of questions, wanting to know why he never went out anymore, why he was being so weird all the time. Jack would get so annoyed with them. It was none of their business what he was doing at home alone at night. Didn't they all have lives of their own to think about?! He reasoned that they were all just very immature souls who didn't know how to spend time alone with their thoughts, enjoying their own company, but sometimes, when he was truly alone with yet another long evening stretching out ahead of him, Jack would feel a deep longing for someone he could share his thoughts with. But how could he possibly let someone else in after so many toxic relationships, and intimate connections that had emotionally suffocated him or simply hadn't allowed him to be himself.

Jack wasn't sure he was ready to trust anyone again. He felt uncomfortable in company, even when he craved it. He was always expecting the next heartbreak and wondering where it would come from and who was about to let him down next. However hard he tried, he just couldn't let go of those old wounds and let-downs, and in his loneliest moments he would admit to himself that he was angry about the past and unwilling to give anyone an opportunity to hurt him again.

He knew it wasn't natural to be this way and that there might be something slightly unhealthy about his behaviour and attitude, but Jack was a very deeply disappointed person. He was suspicious of everyone and everything.

He would constantly fantasise about having a wide circle of great friends and a fun life-partner who would see him for who he was and maybe even bring him out of himself. Sometimes he would imagine himself accepting the next social offer or invitation that came his way. He even picture himself getting dressed to go out, feeling excited as he left the house, not knowing what exhilarating and enriching events lay ahead of him, but when the next phone call came asking him out to a group dinner or a party, his chest would tighten, his heart would start racing and he would find himself panicking, freezing and almost automatically saying he was too busy or had a deadline to meet, or making some other excuse that would let him off the hook once again.

Then, once his friend had finally accepted his excuse and he was truly free to continue his life of lonely but blissfully predictable seclusion, he would feel a mixture of giddy relief, tinged with complete and utter disappointment in himself. He would be happy that his heart palpitations had subsided but there would always be a nagging sense at the back of his mind that life would be unbearable if it was always going to be this way. Yet despite his frustration, he just couldn't seem to figure out what he was afraid of, or why he was letting it get in the way of his happiness. When was his life ever going to begin again? When was he ever going to just let go of the past and allow himself to re-join the human race?

Being a writer, Jack was almost free to become a total recluse and he often convinced himself that this was simply the way it had to be for people in his profession. Of *course* he wanted to go out and have fun like everyone else, but his job just wouldn't allow him to..

If Jack worked steadily on healing his wounded heart chakra, he would experience a gradual opening to new experiences. He could finally begin to take small steps to release his social anxiety. He might begin by tentatively sharing some of his thoughts and feeling with his closest friends and then, encouraged by their kind and understanding responses, he might find himself thinking more clearly about which types of social activity he would find most comfortable. He might enjoy a trip to the cinema with just one or two friends. With something else to concentrate on, he might find it easier to allow himself to be in company without feeling a great deal of anxiety or pressure to interact with large groups of people. He might then enjoy discussing the film over a quiet drink and gradually finding his way back into socialising in a calmer and more gentle way. He might gradually find himself worrying less about what people thought of him and seeing a much wider perspective on life, wisely observing that other people did indeed have a range of other preoccupations and concerns in life. With this new, wider perspective, he might even find himself reaching out to help his friends with their concerns or to listen as they shared their problems. He might not find an instant cure for his panic attacks, but his symptoms would become less acute as he began to embrace the idea of going out for walks in the countryside, where he could inhale the healing qualities found in nature. He might find that he had more in common with his friends than he realised and that, as the song says, "everybody hurts sometimes."

By committing to deep and lasting healing, he might find himself developing more compassion for others and generally feeling less afraid to take chances, and despite his deadlines and work pressures, he might even begin to find more enjoyable ways of living, working and being in the world. In time, he might find himself absent-mindedly checking dating sites or noticing attractive women while he was out socialising, and after enough positive social experiences, he might gradually rebuild his trust, just enough to let someone in – someone with whom he could open up and share his heart.

18.1 Healing and Maintenance of the Heart Chakra

So how do you know if your heart chakra is blocked or out of balance? If you answer yes to three or more of the questions below, it's highly likely that it is.

1. Do you feel it's necessary to isolate yourself from others in order to feel safe?

2. Are you afraid to let someone in emotionally, and does even the idea of developing an intimate relationship cause you to panic?

3. Do you sometimes have strange sensations or tightness in the chest area?

4. Do you tend to be more withdrawn than before, when in company, taking a back seat and allowing others to do all the talking and socialising?

5. Do you often feel desperately lonely even though you seem to have chosen to live as a semi-recluse?

If your heart chakra is blocked, out of balance or in need of healing, try some of the remedies and practices below to help bring it back into balance and restore harmony and wellbeing.

Meditation for Healing the Heart Chakra

Close your eyes and sit in a comfortable position with your feet planted firmly on the floor.

Breathe deeply and visualise white light streaming down from above and creating a thick, protective energy bubble around you.

Place both hands on your heart and breathe deeply into the chest area.

Visualise a rich, deep green light streaming down into the heart chakra from your hands.

If you have trouble visualising, simply close your eyes and repeat the following words:

Rich, deep, green light, rich, deep, green light. Continue repeating these words mentally and silently, until you're able to believe in, and possibly even see, glimpses or flashes of this deep, forest green light streaming into your heart chakra, healing, cleansing and recharging it with its required colour vibration.

Carry out this meditation for approximately twenty minutes or until you feel peaceful and re-energised. Making a regular habit of working on each of your chakras in this way, using the uniquely appropriate chakra colours, will ensure that your chakras remain clear, energised and in perfect balance with each other.

Future Care and Maintenance of the Heart Chakra

As much as time allows, be sure to use this meditation regularly to recharge, heal and balance your heart chakra, but in order keep this chakra whole and healthy and your outlook positive and bright, here are some measures you can take to ensure the ongoing health of this chakra.

Healing Behaviours for Maintaining Good Heart Chakra Health

Begin spending more time in nature, surrounded by greenery and wide-open green spaces. Immerse yourself in the healing vibrations of trees and plants. I often feel that in our highly toxic and inorganic world, filled with metal, glass and pollution, it's only when we take time to connect with the natural world that we can find, heal and recharge ourselves fully. When we absorb the precious life-giving life-force energy generated by the trees, the flowers and the wonderful sights we see on a beautiful country walk, not only do we heal our bodies in the generic sense, we also heal our heart chakras and respiratory organs, by literally allowing the trees to breathe us back into life. As we exhale the carbon-dioxide they need in order to photosynthesise, we inhale the much-needed oxygen they give back to us as a by-product of this process.

But our healing experience in nature goes much deeper into our essential being than this simple biological exchange and occurs on many levels across several dimensions. As we feast on this literal breath of fresh air, we also fill our heart chakras with life, vitality, peace and serenity. At this point, I feel inspired to mention the latest Japanese craze sweeping across Western shores: **Shinrin Yoku**, which translates as 'forest bathing' – the practice of spending time in a forest, walking, breathing, relaxing and allowing the natural world to heal you.

Forest bathing has been said to reduce stress and high blood pressure, improve sleep and even heighten intuition. It should come as no surprise, then, that all the above conditions are present within us when the heart chakra is healthy, clean and energised. When we spend time in a forest, we are literally bathing in precious life-giving oxygen and pranic life-force energy. And the most important colour for the cleansing, healing and effective functioning of the heart chakra... deep forest green.

As well as connecting with the natural world, we can also open our heart chakras by reaching out in service to others. If you have the time and feel so inclined, volunteering to help those less fortunate will allow you to change someone else's life, while also opening your heart to the more compassionate side of your nature.

Using Colour to Heal and Recharge the Heart Chakra

Wear more green and pink shades and tones and introduce these colours in your choice of clothing and furnishings to increase your awareness of them and allow your mind and your energy-field to absorb their vibration as you go about your daily routines.

Crystals for Heart Chakra Cleansing and Balancing

Lie down in a quiet room and place a few cleansed and energised pieces of green aventurine, rose quartz, rhodochrosite, green malachite and/or jade crystals on your heart chakra area for twenty minutes or so. Try this once a week until you get used to the feel of these powerful energies. While you're healing this chakra, you can also carry these stones around with you or wear them on a necklace or bracelet.

Essential Oils for Clearing and healing the Heart Chakra

Massage your chest and arms with gentle love-filled essential oils of rose, frankincense, neroli, melissa, lavender and jasmine. Please remember to always dilute your essential oils with a good quality carrier oil before applying them directly to the skin.

Yoga for Clearing and Healing the Heart Chakra

If you're a yoga practitioner and have no impediments to physical exercise, you might like to try the following yoga poses, to help open, clear and release toxic energy from the heart chakra:

- **Cobra pose**

- **Upward facing dog pose**

- **Fish pose**

- **Camel pose**

Remember that it's always best to study yoga with a qualified instructor, and if you're studying at home, please be gentle with yourself and go at a slow and steady pace that you know you can manage easily. Sometimes we gain the best results from the smallest of movements carried out in just the right way.

See the healing table at the end of this book for a comprehensive cheat sheet on all the tips and techniques that will help you to strengthen each chakra.

Happy Heart Chakra Healing!

19. Finding a Voice: Balancing the Throat Chakra

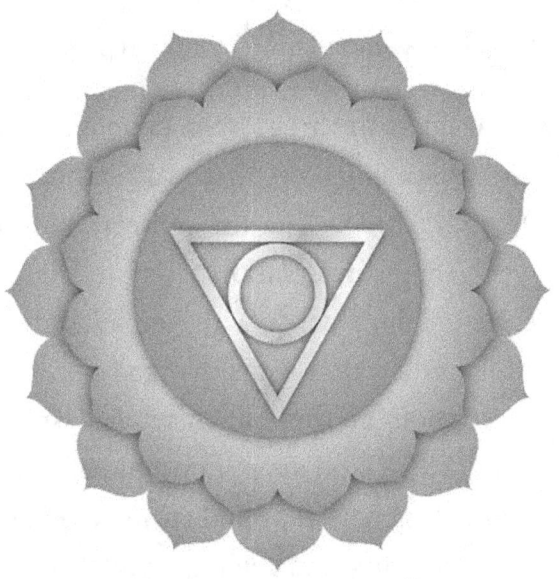

Simone was a quiet and unassuming woman who worked in her local branch of a high street bank. She found her job easy and mostly stress-free, but she suspected that this was probably because she'd never really challenged herself or put herself forward when opportunities for advancement had arisen. Although she had been working at the bank longer than any of her colleagues, she would constantly find herself taking a back seat in meetings and getting frustrated with herself later, knowing that she could have contributed so much more.

Simone's line manager was puzzled by her seeming lack of ambition, but Simone felt bewildered about how to communicate her true desires. Most of the time, she wasn't even sure what they were. Over the years, she had seen many new colleagues arrive at the bank and rise quickly through the ranks.

Most of her seniors had once been her equals, and she was surrounded by young ambitious types who were destined to move up the ladder while she stood there watching silently and unassumingly, as life went rushing by at warp speed.

Simone shared a flat with three other people and would often find herself doing washing up that wasn't hers rather than speaking up for herself. She loathed confrontation of any kind and shied away from conversations that might allow her to reach more equal arrangements with her flatmates. Inside she would be seething when they later thanked her for doing their share of the household chores but instead of speaking up for herself, she would shrug and say, "no problem." It was so much easier than formulating her ideas and sitting down with them to discuss her true thoughts and feelings. She would rather find somewhere else to live than be pressured into speaking up. She would rather find a new job than answer any more uncomfortable questions about why she had been stuck in the same role for over twenty years.

Simone's boyfriend was always encouraging her to stand up for herself and ask for what she wanted and deserved, but when she tried to, the words would simply get stuck in her throat. None of her friends or family members could understand what was keeping her from progressing in life. She was a great thinker and organiser, she was hard-working, fastidious about details and could probably have done everyone else's job as well as her own without even breaking a sweat. But if she was ever asked to give a presentation or greet a visiting client, she would do exactly that – break out in a cold, clammy sweat, all over. Just the thought of standing up and giving any kind of talk or presentation would have her feeling faint and nauseous and recalling memories of being told at school that her ideas were weird, or her voice was squeaky.

She once briefly joined a local gospel choir, hoping it would cure her of her fear of expressing herself in public, and for a while she had impressed herself with her growing confidence, and had even found that the sound of her own voice was actually not that bad! It had a richness and depth that she hadn't known she'd possessed, and she even began to imagine herself developing into a confident singer and, eventually, a more confident speaker. She sang perfectly in tune and loved the sound of her voice blending with other voices and creating a sound she could be proud of. The horrible sore throats and swollen glands that had plagued her since childhood began to disappear and her confidence was beginning to grow in other areas as well. She would find herself occasionally making tentative suggestions at work, as long as she could make them in private, to her sympathetic line manager.

Her line manager, of course responded positively to her well-thought-out suggestions and asked her why she had never considered asking for a promotion, and despite the crazy sensation of butterflies in her stomach, for a while she actually began to give the suggestion some serious consideration.

Simone had begun to heal her throat chakra issues by following her inner guidance to begin singing – one of the most wonderfully freeing and fun ways to approach this healing.

However, when she was asked to take her first solo for the choir's next upcoming public performance, she felt her old fears returning. It was too soon. She just wasn't ready. She knew in her heart that despite her newfound vocal confidence, this was just too much of a big leap, but she pushed herself and took a chance.

On the night of her first performance, Simone was a nervous wreck and she wondered how she was ever going to force herself to get to the venue, but she also hated letting people down, so she persevered and forced herself out through the front door regardless of her fears.

On the way to the performance, she could feel her throat tightening in a very unpleasant way. It was just like being back at school and preparing for another day of ridicule about the sound of her voice. "Squeaky Simone, Squeaky Simone" echoed loudly in her ears, as she opened her mouth to sing the first line of "Oh Happy Day" only to find with horror that nothing more than a pitch-less, toneless and truly unpleasant squeak emerged from her taut but trembling lips.

For the next few months Simone was inconsolable about the performance and despite the reassurances of her choir leader, she never found the courage to return to the hobby that had made her so happy for a while. At work, she returned to being quiet, unassuming and subdued and at home things were worse than even. She became unable to even fully express her feelings to her boyfriend, simply insisting that she didn't want to talk about anything that was happening in her life. For the time being, her healing was postponed, life carried on as it had been before, and Simone remained voiceless, frustrated and unhappy.

If Simone chose to continue working on her throat chakra, she would find that her confidence in her voice would gradually return. In time, she would not only begin taking risks in communicating but might also develop the inner confidence to take other kinds of risks, wisely viewing her perceived failures as learning experiences and opportunities to grow. Her voice would eventually grow stronger with proper training and use, and she would learn not only how to express herself better as a singer and a speaker, but how to express her deepest feelings, wishes and desires as well. In time, she would also find a way to give herself the time, space and freedom to connect with her true nature and life purpose and to discover her highest form of self-expression. She would learn to enjoy speaking up and singing out and might even learn to love the sound of her own voice.

19.1 Healing and Maintenance of the Throat Chakra

So how do you know if your throat chakra is out of balance? If you answer yes to three or more of the questions below, it's highly likely that it is.

1. Do you often have trouble communicating your true feelings, even to close friends, intimate partners and family members?

2. Do you suffer from throat complains and sudden flare-ups of laryngitis when asked to speak or sing in public?

3. Do you hold back from saying what you truly think and feel for the sake of keeping the peace, whatever the personal cost?

4. Do you lack confidence in your ideas and experience anxiety when asked your opinions in public?

5. Are you longing to express yourself in a career that feels more true and real to you, but always lacking the confidence and authority to make changes in your life?

If your throat chakra is blocked, out of balance or in need of healing, try some of the remedies and practices below to help bring it back into balance and restore harmony and wellbeing.

Meditation for Healing the Throat Chakra

Close your eyes and sit in a comfortable position with your feet planted firmly on the floor.

Breathe deeply and visualise white light streaming down from above and creating a thick, protective energy bubble around you.

Place both hands on your throat and breathe deeply into this area.

Visualise a soft cornflower blue light streaming down into the throat from your hands.

If you have trouble visualising, simply close your eyes and repeat the following words:

Soft, blue light, soft, blue light. Continue repeating these words mentally and silently, until you're able to believe in, and possibly even see, glimpses or flashes of this beautiful, soothing cornflower blue light streaming into your throat chakra, healing, cleansing and recharging it with its true colour vibration.

Carry out this meditation for approximately twenty minutes or until you feel peaceful, recharged and re-energised. Making a regular habit of working on each of your chakras in this way, using the uniquely appropriate chakra colours, will ensure that all your chakras are clear, energised and in perfect balance with each other.

Future Care and Maintenance of the Throat chakra

As much as time allows, be sure to use this meditation to regularly recharge, heal and balance your throat chakra, but in order keep this chakra whole and healthy and your outlook positive and bright, here are some measures you can take to ensure the ongoing health of this chakra.

Healing Behaviours for Maintaining Good Throat Chakra Health

Start by using your voice in interesting and unusual ways, which might not be entirely familiar to you. Awaken this chakra with singing, chanting, humming or by simply laughing a lot more. As you break through years of stagnant programming with the help of these new habits, begin to experiment with speaking your truth in previously difficult situations.

Using Colour to Heal and Recharge the Throat Chakra

Wear more blue tones and include more blue features in your furnishings and fixtures, to increase your awareness of this peaceful colour and allow it to have a subtle influence on your mind and energy-field as you go about your daily routines.

Crystals for Throat Chakra Cleansing and Balancing

Lie down in a quiet room and place a few cleansed and charged pieces of lapis lazuli, sodalite, labradorite or amazonite crystals on your throat chakra area for twenty minutes or so. Try this once a week until you get used to the feel of these powerful energies. While you're healing this chakra, you can also carry these stones around with you or wear them on a necklace or bracelet.

Essential Oils for Clearing and healing the Throat chakra

Massage your throat and upper chest with peppermint, lavender or clary sage essential oil. Please remember to always dilute your essential oils with a good quality carrier oil before applying them to the skin.

Yoga for Clearing and Healing the Throat Chakra

If you're a yoga practitioner and have no impediments to physical exercise, you might like to try the following yoga poses to help you to open, clear and release stagnant energy from the throat chakra area:

- **Plow pose**

- **Upward plank pose**

- **Bridge**

- **Fish pose**

- **Child's pose**

Remember that it's always best to study yoga with a qualified instructor, and if you're studying at home, please be gentle with yourself and go at a slow and steady pace that you know you can handle. Sometimes we gain the best results from the smallest of movements carried out in the right way.

See the healing table at the end of this book for a comprehensive cheat sheet on all the tips and techniques that will help you to strengthen each chakra.

Happy throat chakra healing!

20. Darkest Before Dawn: Balancing the Third Eye Chakra

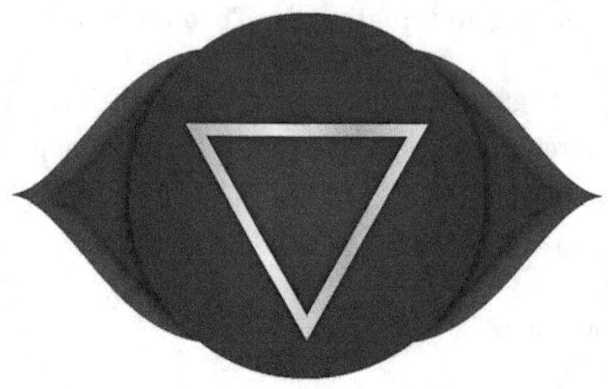

Daniel was a kind, hard-working man who was the head of a company that was responsible for organising wellness retreats around the world. He was passionate about his work and put himself under enormous pressure to create wonderfully uplifting courses and life-changing packages that would bring healing, education and rejuvenation. He loved his work, he ate, slept and breathed it, but he very rarely gave himself a holiday. His work was everything and everything was work. Even while travelling abroad with his family, he was always on the lookout for the next wonderful healing modality, health craze or interesting accommodation and retreat spaces.

Despite his attention to detail, Daniel often found himself making silly mistakes, particularly when required to use his intuition to make decisions about business partners and new joint ventures. He would often experience intense headaches and feelings of paranoia whenever the time came to make a new decision. How could he possibly trust his intuition when he had made so many mistakes, and how could he even run a wellness business when he was clearly so out of touch with his own sense of wellness!

He often felt like a fraud and believed everyone else felt the same way about him. He would torture himself with these thoughts at night and often had nightmares about people chasing him and trying to get at him - business competitors, leaders of enterprises he'd dealt with in the past and an angry parade of clients who felt his retreats hadn't actually been all that life-changing at all! Clients who probably wanted their money back. Sometimes, last thing at night, he would see their faces and would attempt to block them out by listening to subliminal programming audios. But their voices were always stronger and their faces more insistent.

Daniel was beyond frustrated. He seemed unable to tune in to the positive and encouraging sources of guidance he had connected with at the beginning of his journey. Life had been much simpler then – just him and his wife in their cosy yurt, organising weekend meditation retreats and living on raw vegan food. He'd always been so intuitive then. It was almost as if he'd been able to see into the future - a clear road ahead where everything he visualised was a perfectly logical and lucid next step from everything he'd created so far. Now, when he closed his eyes and tried to gain clarity and insights about the future, there was just a cloudy haze of faces.

Despite Daniel's success, there was a sense of pointlessness to everything he did, and there were times when he truly believed his work didn't actually make that much of a difference to anyone. Business was booming but what did it all mean anyway?! The momentum was gone, the sense of purpose was dwindling, and he had no clear sense of direction regarding how to proceed or what to create next, and why. His headaches were becoming unbearable, and his sinuses were constantly having fare-ups and becoming infected, but his doctor could find nothing else wrong with him and put it all down to stress and overwork. He advised Daniel to take up meditation and treat himself to a holiday..or maybe even spend a few weeks at a health retreat...

If Daniel took the time to work on healing and releasing the blockages in his third eye chakra, he would gradually find himself becoming calmer and more confident in his decision-making abilities. He would develop a greater sense of seeing around corners and imagining what results could come from any planned actions he might take, and he would give himself time and space to consider his options more deeply, taking one step at a time in the execution of his plans. When circumstances changed, he would stop, breathe and give himself time to adapt to the changes, gradually becoming more trusting, flexible and open to redirection. He would gradually develop an inner conviction that no matter what choices we make, life is a journey of self-discovery and things ultimately always work out for the highest and best good.

With regular and consistent work, he would soon begin to feel more in touch with divine sources of guidance and might also experience an increase in his intuitive abilities. In connecting with divine, higher wisdom, he would also begin to regain a deeper sense of purpose. In learning to trust his intuition again, he would begin to envision exciting possible timelines, goals, plans and potential futures, which he would execute with skilful planning and a sense of fun. Healing and Maintenance of the Third Eye Chakra

So how do you know if your third eye chakra is out of balance? If you answer yes to three or more of the questions below, it's highly likely that it is.

1. Do you feel you've become unable to trust your intuition when making decisions?

2. Do you sometimes feel you have lost sight of your initial vision and intentions in starting a career or project or committing to a life purpose?

3. Do you find it difficult to sleep, haunted by strange dreams and fearful visions?

4. Do you experience frequent headaches caused by fear, stress and indecision?

5. Do you worry about the future but feel strangely disconnected from it, unable to make decisions based on likely future outcomes – just flailing around in the dark and making a succession of poor choices? Do you sometimes feel paranoid?

If your third eye chakra is blocked, out of balance or in need of clearing and healing, try some of the remedies and practices below to help bring it back into balance and restore harmony and wellbeing.

Meditation for Healing the Third Eye Chakra

Close your eyes and sit in a comfortable position with your feet planted firmly on the floor.

Breathe deeply and visualise white light streaming down from above and creating a thick, protective energy bubble around you.

Place both hands on your heart and breathe deeply into the throat area.

Visualise a deep indigo light streaming down into the throat from your hands.

If you have trouble visualising, simply close your eyes and repeat the following words:

Deep indigo light, deep purple light, deep indigolight, deep purple light. Continue repeating these words mentally and silently, until you're able to believe in, and possibly even see, flashes of deep purple and deep indigo light streaming into your third eye chakra, healing, cleansing and recharging it with an influx of its true colour vibration.

Carry out this meditation for approximately thirty minutes or until you feel peaceful, recharged and re-energised. Making a regular habit of working on each of your chakras in this way, using the uniquely appropriate chakra colours, will ensure that all your chakras are clear, energised and in perfect balance with each other.

Ongoing Maintenance of the Third Eye Chakra

As much as time allows, be sure to use this meditation regularly to recharge, heal and balance your third eye chakra, but in order keep this chakra whole and healthy and your outlook positive and bright, here are some measures you can take to ensure the ongoing health of this chakra.

Healing Behaviours for Maintaining Good Third Eye Chakra Health

Don't be afraid to be an individual, walking your own quirky and unique path through life. Trying to fit in with the rest of society is a sure way to shut down your intuition and cloud your inner vision. Be true to yourself and trust in your own unique vision.

Using Colour to Heal and Recharge the Third Eye Chakra

Wear more deep indigo and purple tones and use them in your furnishings and fixtures to increase your awareness of them and allow your mind and your energy-field to absorb their powerful vibrations as you go about your daily routines.

Crystals for Third Eye Chakra Cleansing and Balancing

Lie down in a quiet room and place a few cleansed and charged pieces of celestite, azurite, selenite or angelite crystals on your third eye and brow area for twenty minutes or so. Try this once a week until you get used to the feel of these powerful energies. While you're healing this chakra, you can also carry these stones around with you or wear them on a necklace or bracelet.

Essential Oils for Clearing and Healing the Third Eye Chakra

Massage your third eye with marjoram, lavender, frankincense and bay oils. Please remember to always dilute your essential oils with a good quality carrier oil before applying them to the skin.

Yoga for Clearing and Healing the Third Eye Chakra

If you're a yoga practitioner and have no impediments to physical exercise, you might like to try the following yoga poses to help open, clear and release stagnant energy in the third eye area:

- **Downward facing dog**

- **Child's pose**

- **Standing half forward bend**

Remember that it's always best to study yoga with a qualified instructor. If you're studying at home, please be gentle with yourself and go at a slow and steady pace that you know you can handle; sometimes we gain the best results from the smallest of movements executed in just the right way.

See the healing table at the end of this book for a comprehensive cheat sheet on all the tips and techniques that will help you to strengthen each chakra.

Happy third eye chakra healing!

21. A Ball of Confusion: Balancing the Crown Chakra

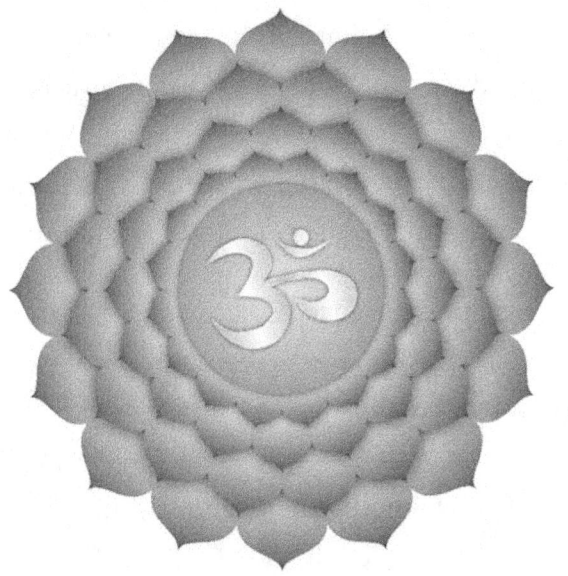

Adriana had always been a very sporadic sleeper; in fact, she would often joke with her friends that she never really slept at all. As a result of her insomnia, she was always fuzzy-headed and utterly drained. No matter how hard she tried, she just couldn't seem to fall asleep at a decent time, and when she did, she felt restless and half-awake until the early hours of the morning. Then, of course, at 5 am, just an hour before her alarm would go off, she'd fall into a deep, almost somnambulistic sleep.

Adriana's inability to sleep dominated her life. It dramatically impaired her thinking ability during the day, and the copious amounts of coffee she drank just to remain conscious would have an irritatingly slow impact, keeping her barely awake in the afternoons when she needed it most and transforming her into a snappy, hyperactive lunatic in the late evening hours. She wandered through life in a perpetual haze of sleeplessness, irritability, confusion, indecision and more sleeplessness. She could never think clearly enough to make decisions, so life just sort of happened around her. She was often accused of being inconsistent in her behaviour and opinions, but it wasn't so much a case of her not knowing what she thought about things, she just never had the presence of mind to even think!

At work, she was often accused of not concentrating – her mind would wander so easily. Projects were never completed on time, assignments were usually handed in way past their deadline, files went missing, phone calls went mysteriously unmade, emails remained woefully unanswered, but she was mostly cooperative and easy to get along with at work and was forgiven each time. And, each time, she promised herself she would get some sleep and do better in future.

Every time it happened; she knew she needed to get help, but the opportunity somehow never came. She was always behind on work, behind on sleep and behind on generally thinking things through! She could never set any goals or stick to a timetable and after a while, the long nights spent poring over books, tables and graphs, desperately trying to catch up on absurdly late assignments would give her headaches and make her eyes twitch.

At weekends, she was too depressed to go out anywhere and on Monday mornings, not only would she still be exhausted from the previous week, she would also be utterly despondent about dragging herself out of bed to face the week that lay ahead.

As Adriana's problems with insomnia persisted, she found herself becoming forgetful: leaving her belongings on buses, losing essential notes, and minutes from essential meetings, forgetting people's names; the list of misdemeanours was seemingly endless. Her ability to think clearly was becoming increasingly impaired and there were many occasions when she would walk into a room and be absolutely convinced that her colleagues had been discussing her ineptitude.

Her moods became changeable and she became highly sensitive to loud noises and physical contact and unwilling to listen to the thoughts and ideas of others. What was the point, she reasoned; they all wanted her fired anyway. Some of them were probably even trying to sabotage her. When she began to see strange shapes and colours before her eyes, she took a visit to her doctor who prescribed anti-depressants and told her she needed some time off. It was at this point that she decided it was probably time to take a different approach.

If Adriana spent some of her time off healing her crown chakra, she would begin to feel generally more at peace within herself. By clearing and healing this chakra she would become more able to sense and receive divine love, light, wisdom and comfort and would, as a result, gradually begin to feel less tired and confused. Consciously or unconsciously, she would begin to feel the love of a divine higher consciousness surrounding her. She would feel less alone in the world, and with prolonged and continuous healing and meditation, she would learn to see herself, her life and even her colleagues through the eyes of divine love and light.

If she persisted in this healing journey and developed a regular, long-term meditation practice, she would finally release the anxieties that had caused her to disconnect from divinity and place her focus on the hard, cold realities of material existence. In this way, she would allow herself to relax on every level, perhaps clearing her mind of worry, and healing her sleeplessness once and for all, knowing that she is loved, all is love and there is absolutely nothing to worry about.Healing and Maintenance of the Crown Chakra

So how do you know if your crown chakra is out of balance? If you answer yes to three or more of the questions below, it's highly likely that it is.

1. Do you suffer from long-term insomnia and episodes of dizziness?

2. Do you lack concentration and find it hard to focus on seeing long-term projects and tasks through to completion?

3. Do you have frequent headaches focused on the area at the very top of the head?

4. Do you feel a lack of faith in, and perhaps even anger towards a higher power?

5. Do you feel alone, disconnected and abandoned by God and your angels and guides, or a general disconnection from the spiritual side of life?

If your crown chakra is blocked, out of balance or in need of healing, try some of the remedies and practices below to help bring it back into balance and restore harmony and wellbeing.

21.1 Meditation for Healing the Crown Chakra

Close your eyes and sit in a comfortable position with your feet planted firmly on the floor.

Breathe deeply and visualise white light streaming down from above and creating a thick, protective energy bubble around you.

Place both hands over your crown chakra and breathe deeply.

Visualise pure white light streaming down into the top of your head through your hands.

If you have trouble visualising, simply close your eyes and repeat the following words:

Pure white light, cleanse and reunite me with the divine, violet flame cleanse and heal. Continue repeating these words mentally and silently, until you feel able to believe in, and possibly even see glimpses of pure white light and violet light streaming into your crown chakra, healing, cleansing and energising it with these essential colour vibrations.

Carry out this meditation for approximately twenty minutes, or until you feel peaceful, and re-energised. Making a regular habit of working on each of your chakras in this way, using the uniquely appropriate chakra colours, will ensure that all your chakras are clear, energised and in perfect balance with each other.

Future Care and Maintenance of the Crown Chakra

As much as time allows, be sure to use this meditation regularly to recharge, heal and balance your throat chakra, but in order keep this chakra whole and healthy and your outlook positive and bright, here are some measures you can take to ensure the ongoing health of this chakra.

Healing Behaviours for Maintaining Good Crown Chakra Health

Practise walking silently in nature or begin a regular meditation practice. As you spend more time reconnecting with your higher self and your inner truth, you will gradually be rewarded with feelings of restored faith, inner strength and comfort. In time, your divine connection will return, along with your memory of who you came into this lifetime to be. With regular practice, you will return to an understanding that no matter how severe the separation from the divine may seem to be at times, we are never, ever alone.

Using Colour to Heal and Recharge the Crown Chakra

Wear more white and violet tones and include more of these colours in your home décor and furnishings, so that your mind and energy-field will absorb their finer vibration as you go about your daily routines.

Crystals for Crown Chakra Cleansing and Balancing

Lie down in a quiet room and place clean and energised pieces of amethyst, clear quartz and herkimer diamond crystals on your pillow, just above the crown chakra area for twenty minutes or so. Try this once a week until you get used to the feel of these powerful energies. While you're healing this chakra, you can also carry these stones around with you or wear them on a necklace or bracelet.

Essential Oils for Clearing and Healing the Crown Chakra

Massage your crown chakra with lavender, spikenard, lotus, rose, cedarwood, lemon and/or rosemary essential oils. Please remember to always dilute your essential oils with a good quality carrier oil before applying them to the skin.

Yoga for Clearing and Healing the Crown Chakra

If you're a yoga practitioner and have no impediments to physical exercise, you might like to try the following yoga poses to help open, clear and release stagnant energy from the crown chakra.

- **Resting pose**

- **Tree pose**

- **Half lotus**

Remember that it's always best to study yoga with a qualified instructor, and if you're studying at home, please be gentle with yourself and go at a slow and steady pace that you know you can handle. Sometimes we gain the best results from the smallest of movements carried out in just the right way. See the healing table at the end of this book for a comprehensive cheat sheet on all the tips and techniques that will help you to strengthen each chakra.Happy crown chakra healing!

22. Chakra Yoga: Yoga for Clearing and Balancing the Chakras

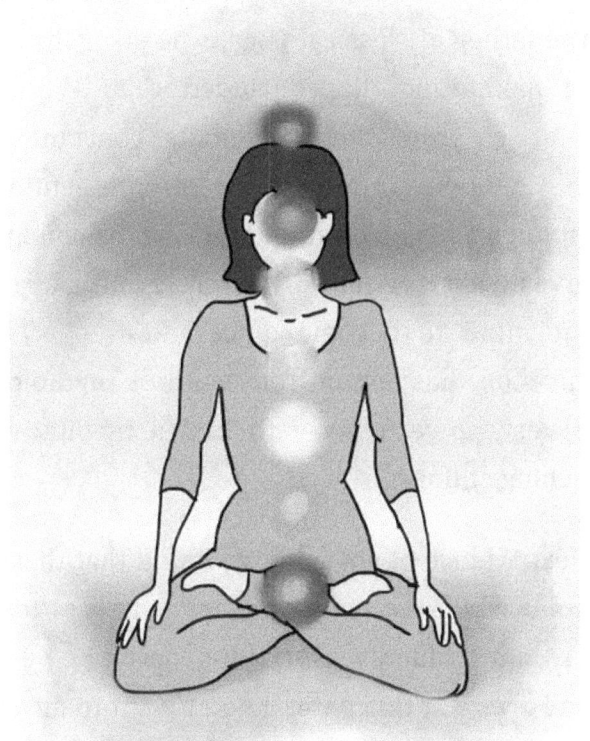

Anyone who has read or researched information on chakra healing will have come across chakra yoga at some point in their journey. If this is your chosen way of clearing and healing your chakras, you might simply find this book useful for understanding which chakras to focus on in your yoga practice.

My focus throughout this book, so far, has been on the influence of chakras in daily life and how to clear, heal, shield and protect them with life-force energy, love, light and intention.

However, here are just a few of my thoughts and experiences regarding why yoga is such a powerful tool for maintaining good chakra health.

Yoga is a kind of meditation extended into physicality. When Patanjali, the father of classical yoga, was struggling to become still during meditation, he concluded that a great deal of distraction arises from the body - its constant needs and restlessness. So, he began to experiment with gentle stretching at the beginning of his meditation sessions, believing that if the body was given what it required, it would eventually settle down, allowing the mind to become quiet and free of distraction. Whether this story has arisen from truth or mythology, yoga is certainly a very powerful way to find a meditative place of deeply enriching stillness.

In my own experience of yoga, I have found that there is always a certain point when the body does indeed seem to release its restlessness, and suddenly everything becomes very still and quiet. When I arrive at this point, I don't want to move or speak; I don't care what's happening in the class or what I'm supposed to be doing next. I just want to be quiet and still. This is one of the reasons I prefer to practice at home – to have freedom to obey the stillness.

As an intuitive, energy practitioner and psychic, I believe that this is the point when the chakras have all been cleared by the dynamic movement of prana, chi or ki, which yoga facilitates. Yoga creates a powerful flushing movement of prana through the entire energy system, including the chakras, and effectively cleanses the body (or bodies), heart, mind, spirit, soul and chakras, and when the chakras are clear and balanced, we become quiet, calm and clear-headed.

If you find this subject interesting and would like to find out more about yoga as a tool for spiritual awakening and development, you might want to do some research on chakra yoga, kundalini yoga and/or kundalini awakenings.

23. The Third Eye Chakra & Psychic Awareness

Most people, if asked which chakra they find the most fascinating will probably say the third eye chakra because of its association with psychic awareness. So, it seems only right to add a quick note on the subject and share a few tips for awakening this chakra. As a responsible teacher of psychic development, I highly recommend that you find yourself a skilled guide or mentor, if you wish to explore psychic development in more depth and detail, but here are a few tips for enhancing your awareness of this chakra and increasing your psychic and spiritual awareness.

- Develop a practice of daily meditation and keep a meditation journal for noting down any new insights or visions you receive. The more frequently you do this practice, the better the results you'll see. If you make it a daily practice, you are sure to see results over time, so don't give up if nothing happens in the first few weeks and it takes a while for your mind to settle down.

- Use bay and lavender oil to increase your awareness in this area. Mix one or two drops of each oil in 10 ml of carrier oil and carefully dab a small drop of the mixture over your third eye and crown chakras before you begin to meditate.

- Learn to become comfortable with silence and make a regular practice of sitting quietly for ten to twenty minutes whenever you have a problem or question.

When you emerge from the silence, write down any solutions that emerged from that silent space. This way, you'll have a record of successes to look back on when you become doubtful. The more you trust your psychic self to bring you the answers to your most pressing problems, the stronger your psychic gift will become.

- Wear azurite and amethyst crystals to increase your psychic awareness and selenite, celestite and angelite to help you to connect with your angels, guides and ascended master teachers. They will guide you to work from the purest motivations and ensure that the insights you receive will be gentle, loving, healing and wise.

24. Comprehensive Chakra Healing Chart

Chakra	Crystals	Essential Oils	Supportive Behaviours	Yoga Positions
Root Chakra	Red jasper, red carnelian, garnet, bloodstone	Benzoin, cedarwood, patchouli,	Pampering and extreme self-care, tree-hugging, walking on the earth	Cat pose, wide-legged forward bend pose, locust pose
Sacral Chakra	Orange carnelian, citrine, tiger's eye	Orange, neroli, ginger, cinnamon	Take up a creative hobby, be more explorative and spontaneous, learn to ask for and accept help	Full boat pose, cobra, bound angle pose, pelvic tilt
Solar Plexus Chakra	Manipura	Lemon, clary sage, peppermint, fennel	Become more observant in relationships, practice more self-love, develop good boundaries, learn to say no	Bow pose, fish pose, salute to the sun, half lord of the fishespose
Heart Chakra	Rhodochrosite, rose quartz, green aventurine, jade	Rose, jasmine, rosewood, Melissa	Spend time in nature – forest bathing, become a volunteer, develop compassions, develop counselling skills	Cobra pose, downward-facing dog pose, camel pose
Throat Chakra	Lapis lazuli, sodalite, amazonite	Peppermint, lavender, clary sage	Sing, chant, hum and practice using your voice in different ways, learn how to lovingly and assertively express your true feelings	Plow pose, upward plank, Bridge pose, fish pose, child's pose
Third Eye Chakra	Azurite, selenite, celestite, angelite, amethyst	Marjoram, lavender, frankincense, bay	Practice daily meditation and journaling, trust your individuality and your unique vision, take time off when you need to	Downward facing dog Child's pose Standing half forward bend
Crown Chakra	Lotus, spikenard, rose, cedarwood, rosemary	The top of the head	Meditation, chanting, yoga, channelling, walking meditation, prayer	Resting pose Tree pose Half lotus

www.ingramcontent.com/pod-product-compliance
Lightning Source LLC
Chambersburg PA
CBHW072141280526
45788CB00002B/737